W9-CDY-524

INFORMATICS FOR HEALTHCARE PROFESSIONALS

INFORMATICS FOR HEALTHCARE PROFESSIONALS

Kathleen M. Young, MA, RNC
Western Michigan University
Kalamazoo, Michigan

 F. A. DAVIS COMPANY • Philadelphia

F. A. Davis Company
1915 Arch Street
Philadelphia, PA 19103

Copyright © 2000 by F. A. Davis Company

All rights reserved. This book is protected by copyright. No part of it may be reproduced, stored in a retrieval system, or transmitted in any form or by any means, electronic, mechanical, photocopying, recording, or otherwise, without written permission from the publisher.

Printed in the United States of America

Last digit indicates print number: 10 9 8 7 6

Acquisitions Editor: Joanne DaCunha, RN, MSN
Developmental Editor: Peg Waltner
Production Editor: Jessica Howie Martin
Cover Designer: Eric Dush

As new scientific information becomes available through basic and clinical research, recommended treatments and drug therapies undergo changes. The author(s) and publisher have done everything possible to make this book accurate, up to date, and in accord with accepted standards at the time of publication. The authors, editors, and publisher are not responsible for errors or omissions or for consequences from application of the book, and make no warranty, expressed or implied, in regard to the contents of the book. Any practice described in this book should be applied by the reader in accordance with professional standards of care used in regard to the unique circumstances that may apply in each situation. The reader is advised always to check product information (package inserts) for changes and new information regarding dose and contraindications before administering any drug. Caution is especially urged when using new or infrequently ordered drugs.

Library of Congress Cataloging-in-Publication Data

Young, Kathleen M., 1945–
    Informatics for healthcare professionals / Kathleen M. Young.
        p.; cm.
    Includes bibliographical references and index.
    ISBN 0–8036–0619–2 (pbk.)
    1. Medical informatics. I. Title.
    [DNLM: 1. Medical Informatics. W 26.5 Y73i 2000]
    R858.Y68 2000
    362.1'068—dc21

                                    99–088883

Authorization to photocopy items for internal or personal use, or the internal or personal use of specific clients, is granted by F. A. Davis Company for users registered with the Copyright Clearance Center (CCC) Transactional Reporting Service, provided that the fee of $.10 per copy is paid directly to CCC, 222 Rosewood Drive, Danvers, MA 01923. For those organizations that have been granted a photocopy license by CCC, a separate system of payment has been arranged. The fee code for users of the Transactional Reporting Service is: 8036-0619/00 0 + $.10.

Information management skills are essential to clinical practitioners in all healthcare disciplines. Healthcare is increasingly driven by information; consequently, the delivery of patient care demands effective management of information. Inefficient information handling causes problems for practitioners due to incorrect diagnoses, cumbersome assessment strategies, and inappropriate problem statements; overcoming these deficiencies requires that healthcare professionals, from the beginning of their education, start to understand formal information theory as a supportive discipline. Medicine and nursing have taken the lead in informatics, but since the early 1990s a variety of health professions have explored the use of informatics within their disciplines. The value of information handling to support decision making is becoming increasingly obvious in the clinical areas of medicine, nursing, physician assistant, dentistry, pharmacy, occupational therapy, physical therapy, speech pathology, and social service.

Even though the importance of information management is recognized, most educators do not have the background or expertise to teach informatics, and few texts are available for assistance. Despite its pervasiveness and importance, informatics is an area in which students, practitioners, and educators are uneasy. Much of this unease stems from the relative newness of the discipline and the constant change inherent in it. An emphasis on computer hardware and technology has often taken precedence over understanding the multiple processes of managing the information required for sound decision making. It is important to realize that computers and information systems are just tools. The important concept for students is the fact that they are the information managers of the future. Tools and applications will change over time, but the concepts concerning obtaining the right information at the right time and place and in the right amount do not change.

Informatics for Healthcare Professionals is a mid-level, generic informatics book usable as the primary informatics book in a professional healthcare curriculum. It can be used for an entire informatics course or it can be a supplement, supporting the integration of informatics into an existing curriculum. For the future professionals who are the target audience for this book, the relevance of information handling for practice and for their roles as information management leaders in their disciplines is emphasized.

Informatics education can mean anything from teaching simple computer literacy to training others in how to design a medical records system. Curricular content varies widely from one institution to another. Few topics appear to be covered in all educational programs, and the depth and breadth of coverage of selected topics also vary widely. The topics chosen for this book represent a broad overview of subjects relating to informatics. Separate chapters provide the basic applications of informatics in conceptual theory, evidence-based healthcare, taxonomy, security and confidentiality, and electronic and Web-based tools and telehealth. In addition, the book includes chapters on human factors, the systems cycle, managing change, and managed care.

Human factors, a subject often not explored in other books, is emphasized at the beginning of this book. Designing user-centered devices and systems is paramount to user acceptance, efficiency, and accuracy. Devices that gather, monitor, and disseminate information proliferate in healthcare practice. Professionals knowledgeable in the analysis of human factors are an asset to vendor designers and facility system cycles.

Chapter 9 presents a broad overview of the cycle of an automated system from problem identification, the most neglected yet most important step, to implementation and evaluation. Entry-to-practice graduates are not involved in every aspect of the cycle, but all of them are involved at some point. The more knowledgeable the practitioner, the more successful the implementation.

Change is pervasive in today's environment, and all are affected by it. The implementation of an automated system initiates significant cultural changes. The leaders of the future must be prepared to manage the changes successfully or suffer the failure of system implementation, at great monetary and user acceptance costs.

Chapter 10 deals with the use of data and information in managed care. Managed care cannot exist without automation because it is data dependent. The challenge for each professional discipline is to know what data are used to make managed-care decisions and to ensure that discipline-specific outcome data are available to support practice and provide quality care, as determined by the healthcare provider.

For healthcare professionals to realize the potential of informatics, it must be integrated into educational curricula at the entry-to-practice level and the continuing education level. This book is designed to promote that integration. Each chapter contains pedagogical aids that help the reader learn and apply the information discussed. Learning objectives let the reader know what to expect from each chapter. Chapters begin with a real-life scenario to engage the interest of the student and to set the principles presented in the chapter in a contextual framework. The learning exercises at the end of each chapter engage the student in real-life situations, interviews, observations, and discussions centered on the chapter topics. Each chapter also contains a summary and a list of references. The glossary at the end of the book brings the reader up to date with the vocabulary of healthcare informatics.

The purpose of this book is to inform students of the potential of informatics and challenge them to be visionary leaders in the vital area of managing information to make decisions in their practice. During the 4 years I have taught the Informatics for Healthcare Professionals course, I have seen students enter the course computer phobic and finish it feeling empowered in the world of information. Their knowledge of human factors enlightens them to the fact that clumsiness with computer-driven devices and applications is a result not of personal ineptitude but of poor design. They know how to analyze a proposed automated system, and they understand the potential of an automated cradle-to-grave health record. Although graphics application is not taught during class, students learn how to use it to add polish and credibility to their own classroom presentations, patient teaching, and inservice education. Students taking the class who are already in practice immediately understand the relevance of informatics and take their new knowledge back to their places of work. It is my desire that all students become excited and empowered by the potential of informatics in their practice.

Kathleen M. Young

▶▶▶ Acknowledgments

Writing a textbook is a time-consuming, daunting task that cannot be accomplished without the support and assistance of many people. My heartfelt gratitude is extended to my family and colleagues for their patience, encouragement, and quiet amazement that I would even attempt such an endeavor.

Thoughtful and thorough editing assistance was willingly provided by Dr. Diane Hamilton, Dr. Suzan Olson, and my friend Merry Cotton, who changed many of my passive-voice sentences into acceptable active-voice statements. Reviewers supplied insightful comments and suggestions.

Thank you to the team of people assembled by F. A. Davis who have the skills and expertise to mold this manuscript into a professional product. Editor Joanne DaCunha has been a patient, pleasant, encouraging, and steadying voice throughout the process. Developmental editor Peg Waltner has been my guide and organizer for a year and a half.

Most important, thanks to my husband for his help, love, and steadfast support. His constant belief and encouragement always keep me going.

Kathleen M. Young

DeAnn L. Ambroson, PhD, RN
Assistant Professor
Department of Nursing
Mount Mercy College
Cedar Rapids, Iowa

Mary T. Boylston, RN, MSN,
  CCRN
Assistant Professor
Department of Nursing
Eastern College
St. David's, Pennsylvania

Barbara Jean Gibbons, RN,C
  (Informatics), MSN
Assistant Professor, Nurse
  Educator, Nursing Informatics
  Specialist
State University of New York at
  Stony Brook School of Nursing
Stony Brook, NY
Bassett Healthcare
Cooperstown, New York

Kelly Goudreau, M.NURS, RNC,
  CS, APRN
Associate Professor, Nursing
University of Maine at Fort Kent
Fort Kent, Maine

Ruth Mulvaney, MS, PT
Associate Professor
University of Tennessee
Memphis, Tennessee

Christine Neff, RN, BSN
Practical Nursing Instructor
Mid East Ohio Vocational School
Zanesville, Ohio

Evelyn M. Wills, RN, PhD
Associate Professor
University of Southwestern
  Louisiana
College of Nursing
Lafayette, Louisiana

Tami Hodges Wyatt, RN, MSN,
  PhD(c)
Assistant Professor
College of Health Sciences
Roanoke, Virginia

Jack A. P. Yensen, PhD, RN
Instructor
Nursing Department
Lanagra College
Vancouver, British Columbia,
  Canada

▶▶▶ CONTENTS

12. Telehealth 211
LYNNE M. PATZEK MILLER AND KATHLEEN M. YOUNG

13. Information Becomes Knowledge through Research 235
SUZAN D. OLSON

1

The Information Explosion

LEARNING OBJECTIVES

By the end of this chapter, you will be able to:
▶ Describe the impact of the information explosion on society
▶ Describe the emerging impact, positive and negative, of technology on healthcare management and delivery
▶ Create a vision for the future of healthcare technology

Worried parents bring a small 5-year-old boy to his primary physician's office. The boy seems to have influenza, but is not recovering and is rapidly becoming weaker and less responsive. The physician, realizing that the child is acutely ill, has the office clerk admit the child to the local pediatric unit via a computer system located in the office. Also from the office, the physician orders laboratory and diagnostic tests to be done immediately on the boy's admittance to the hospital. Because the pediatrician's office staff sends the patient's demographic information (name, address, date of birth, allergies, insurance information) online to the hospital's admitting department, the child and his parents report directly to the patient's room on their arrival. The physician assessment that was completed in the office and the child's past medical history are already available on the computer in the patient's room.

As the nurse verbalizes the physical assessment while admitting the child, the assessment is entered electronically into the electronic health record through the voice recognition system. The child is attached to noninvasive monitors that continually record vital information into the electronic record. During the nursing assessment, the child indicates that he ate some berries in the woods behind his grandmother's house. The nurse uses a handheld computer to show him pictures of berries from a pictorial database of poisonous berries indigenous to the region. He selects a picture of berries that look like the ones he ate.

The attending physician at the hospital communicates this information to the primary physician using a pic-tel system, so they are communicating verbally and face-to-face electronically. The pictorial database reveals that the berries contain a particularly virulent poison that causes swift liver failure. From the hospital room, the attending physician searches the most recent literature electronically and discovers a recent journal article about a new treatment for this type of poisoning. The toxicologist in Europe who wrote the article is contacted through the electronic pic-tel/voice system. After the physician reveals the details of the situation, the researcher verifies that the experimental treatment may be effective in this instance if it is begun within 48 hours of the poison's ingestion. The conversation is stored and sent to the primary physician's office to be reviewed at the earliest opportunity.

Again using the pic-tel system that automatically dials the desired connection, the two local physicians confer concerning the results of the literature search and the conversation with the researcher. The primary physician follows the child's vital signs and the laboratory results from the office computer workstation across town from the hospital. As the child's vital signs and blood work indicate a rapid decline in the child's condition, the two physicians decide to initiate the experimental European treatment. The treatment quickly reverses the liver failure, and the child recovers. All of this is done in less than 24 hours.

This scenario is not especially futuristic. All of the technology described has been available for several years, and organizations throughout the global healthcare delivery system are investigating and implementing information systems for information retrieval, documentation, and decision making. The recovery of this child was dependent on the efficient **management and processing of information**. The management and processing of information to support decision making in a healthcare practice is a basic necessity in today's complex and rapidly changing world. The people and organizations that are knowledgeable in this area are those that are successfully affecting patient outcomes. This scenario describes the world that current healthcare students will encounter in their practice settings. Preparation for entering this technological environment is a necessary component of today's education.

INFORMATION IS IMPORTANT

In the fall of 1996 two economists, James Mirrlees and William Vickery, won the Nobel Prize for economics for their theory of asymmetric information. **Asymmetric information** refers to a situation in which both sides do not have the same facts. The buyer of a piece of real estate or a car, for example, does not have the same information as the seller. Therefore, the seller has an advantage over the buyer. The buyer must do more research and spend more time and money to gain more information. Awarding the Nobel Prize for the theory of asymmetric information emphasizes the importance of information in all human activity.

IMPACT ON SOCIETY

Cultures worldwide are changing, shifting, and adjusting to the onslaught of **technology** and information. The advances of technology mold and shape daily lives. Instead of communicating face to face, individuals use telephones, leave voice messages, or write e-mail notes. Children's play activities revolve around television and computer games, both of which are continually achieving higher visual resolution and faster speed of transmission. Parents monitor their children's activities, not through a neighborhood watch but through nursery monitors, beepers, cell phones, and Internet cameras at daycare facilities. Telecommunications increasingly support the home office and allow men and women to work at home rather than fighting traffic to commute to the office.

Before telecommunications existed, people communicated through letter writing, an art that was diligently practiced and beautifully exhibited. Before the invention of telephones, television, and computers, friends and neighbors met at the corner store and developed a sense of community. Almost everyone knew his or her neighbors. Now only one-quarter of all Americans know their next-door neighbors. The number of outdoor cafés in Europe is decreasing or the cafés are closing earlier because customers no longer linger over cappuccino to discuss the problems of the world (Swerdlow, 1995). Instead, people meet in virtual "chat rooms" at any time of the day or night and talk with unseen people around the world.

Because of the Internet, a worldwide system that allows computers to communicate with each other, our communities are becoming less intimate and more isolated as individuals earn college credits, begin romances, and engage in gossip electronically. As computer ownership grows, more electronic shopping, bill paying, game playing, and daily reminders are part of daily life. Virtual communities of people who never see, hear, or touch each other are commonplace.

Yet our need to have physical contact and face-to-face interaction with other humans, called "**skin**," has not diminished (Swerdlow, 1995). People still flock to large cities. Shopping malls are crowded even as television and online shopping increases. Industrial parks continue to grow even though more work can be done from the home. People still seek the relationships that come only from being physically with other people.

IMPACT ON TEACHING AND LEARNING

Technology has also changed the way in which learning occurs. Television and computers spawn aliteracy among many people who are unwilling to read anything of substantial length that requires concentration. Brevity, 5-second sound bites, channel surfing, instant gratification, fast-moving images, constant stimulation, and shorter attention spans all reflect today's society. One need only look at *USA Today,* which has become one of the most popular newspapers because of its abbreviated style. The role of the printed word in learning is changing. The intent of university libraries was to allow scholars and would-be scholars to search the tomes of knowledge contained within the library walls. Currently, many books, journals, and newspapers are on line. In the future, all books and journals will be available on line, accessible from home computers. Sales of electronic encyclopedias already exceed sales of printed encyclopedias. Interactive media books offer learning that appeals to every learning style. Sounds, images, and words are all available at the same time. If you are learning a foreign language, you need only click on a word to find the correct pronunciation.

Technology has also changed the methodology of teaching. The creation of universities in the 1900s enabled a large number of students to learn from a single master teacher. This was commonly referred to as learning "at the feet of the master." Teaching and learning at that time followed an oral tradition of communication. The expert's sharing of knowledge with the student happened most efficiently when a large number of students gathered together in one place. Today, with distance learning, a campus with large classrooms is no longer necessary. For example, in Canada the majority of master of business administration (MBA) programs are completely available through distance learning. A master teacher can reach thousands of students around the world in a single session.

To accommodate the change in learning style and to compete for students' attention, teachers have added brevity, movement, color, and technology to their lessons. Elementary school children use graphics presentation software to give presentations in class. Teaching keyboard skills has moved from the middle-school level to the elementary level. Book reports and other large visual assessments at the fourth- and fifth-grade levels are word-processed rather than handwritten. Children learn about the world, both past and present, from software programs instead of, or in addition to, traditional textbooks. To be able to teach children how to use technology, teachers have had to learn how to use it. However, acceptance of new teaching methods is not always quickly embraced and adopted. For example, in the early 1800s an "amazing device" was introduced into the classroom. It was the blackboard. Entire books were written about how to use the blackboard in the classroom. However, early anecdotal reports suggest that teachers were not accepting the new device well. The introduction of new technology into the classroom may create a reaction similar to the introduction of the blackboard.

> Futurist Nicholas Negroponte, a leading authority on the digital revolution, suggests that the information revolution is a reality today and is changing virtually every aspect of our lives, from the way we work and play to the way we communicate and relate to friends and loved ones. He sees programs that "read" news and messages for people with low vision, allow doctors and family to check on frail, homebound persons, even programs to keep your kitchen shelves full. If your refrigerator notices that you are out of milk, it can ask your car to remind you to pick some up on your way home. Your toaster could imprint your toast with the closing price of your favorite stock. [Negroponte] visualized a "daily me," a daily electronic "newspaper" that would mix headline news with stories relating to your life—the people you're going to meet, the places you're going to go.
>
> —Carlson & Glasheen, 1998, pp. 1, 12.

IMPACT ON GOVERNMENT

To remain competitive in a global society, nations must remain receptive to new technology and ideas. Knowledge is power, and information is one source of knowledge that gives power. According to Swerdlow (1995), repressive governments that attempt to control information are finding it increasingly difficult to do so. In China and Burma, government propaganda machines indoctrinated their soldiers to believe that student demonstrators were foreigners or Communists who were trying to take over the country. The soldiers, believing that they were defending their country, opened fire on the student demonstrators. They did not learn until later that the students were fellow countrymen demonstrating for democracy. Romania tried, but failed, to ban the use of typewriters in an attempt to suppress information. Information gained through technology continually assaults authority. Free-flowing information nurtures democracy.

Examples of global communication despite government intervention:
- Popular U.S. TV shows are broadcast via satellite into Iran and Iraq
- Rebels in Mexico's Chiapas state post statements on the Internet

- The work of novelist Pramoedya Anata Toer, which is banned in India, can be read and printed through the Internet

—Swerdlow (1995).

Technology also affects democratic governments. Politicians are perfecting 5-second sound bites and eye-catching visual messages. People want fast, frequent, and abbreviated news rather than lengthy, in-depth analysis. Government officials, academic experts, and policy makers have less effect on decisions, whereas public opinion, informed through various media, plays a larger role in public policy and diplomacy.

IMPACT ON HEALTHCARE

Not only does technology affect society's relationships, government, learning, and teaching, it also has an astounding impact on healthcare. Information technology is part of the daily life of healthcare professionals. Throughout the past three decades, the healthcare literature has described the growing impact of technology on health and human services. According to Steven Smith, Vice President and Editorial Director for Medscape, Inc. (1998), physicians spend 38 percent of their time charting in the medical record. Other healthcare professionals spend this amount of time or more gathering, sharing, or seeking information. Technology assists in managing all stages of information. If information is power, healthcare information affects the power to promote health and wellness. As exemplified in the opening scenario of this chapter, automation enables the practitioner to process information that is accurate, unduplicated, error free, and accessible from remote areas by multiple persons at one time. Information that is rapidly available through technology affects decision making in healthcare. Informed decision makers produce better patient outcomes. Competition has also become a driving force in the pricing and marketing of healthcare. Federal programs like Medicare and Medicaid, health maintenance organizations, and managed-care programs encourage payment methodologies that promote competition. To offer competitive and quality service, information must be readily available to make decisions. Information technology allows this to happen. A leadership survey conducted by *Hospitals & Health Networks* in 1997 reveals that adding information technology is one of the top two goals of hospitals, managed-care organizations, and group practices. To stay competitive in national and international healthcare, the healthcare delivery system, including all allied health professions, must be receptive to new information and ideas.

THE FUTURE OF HEALTHCARE TECHNOLOGY

Methods of using **healthcare technology** in the future are receiving great attention. Forecasters predict that in the year 2000, computers will support and assess the quality of patient care and enhance healthcare professionals' decision making, management, planning, and clinical research. These ideas suggest that computers will not only supplement but also replace many current methods of conceptualizing and delivering healthcare. For example, one vision of the future includes devices called "biosensors" that can read and transmit responses to physical and chemical changes within chronically ill clients such as those with diabetes. The biosensor would monitor blood glucose levels and thus eliminate the need for uncomfortable venipuncture while regulating glucose levels with an implanted insulin pump. Noninvasive technology such as the biosensor reduces discomfort and provides constant, consistent monitoring as opposed to the painful, intermittent monitoring of today that is dependent on client compliance and reporting. Electronic monitoring will also allow people who are chronically ill greater mobility and freedom. They will no longer be restricted to their homes, close to their supplies or to a medical facility. Equipment and supplies will be minimal, with no need to maintain sterility and no danger from bloodborne pathogens. As with most technology, the initial cost may be high, but the long-term costs, both monetary and physiological, will be less than the cost of current methods.

In the future the home, rather than the institution, may be the center for healthcare monitoring. Technologies that support telehealth and telemedicine will create an environment in which home-focused care is cost effective, convenient, and accessible. Instead of entering the healthcare arena through the emergency room, Mr. Jones will e-mail his symptoms to the physician and a personnel status monitor (PSM), developed by SARCOS Corporation, will locate and diagnose his disease. The monitor, a small wristband, will read the surface of Mr. Jones's body, note vital signs, and send the diagnoses and possible treatments to the physician. With a global positioning satellite (GPS), the client's location will also be transmitted to the base site (physician's office). A device such as the envisioned PSM would reduce physician office and emergency room visits. The biosensor and telecommunication combination could also be invaluable for locating a person injured in an accident in a remote area or on a battlefield. SARCOS believes that the PSM is the first of a line of products that will eliminate the waiting room (Kaplan, 1998). As mentioned earlier, however, the need for "skin," personal contact with the care provider, may also be in danger of being lost. Not all diagnosis or counseling is based solely on empirical evidence or on signs and symptoms. The physical demeanor, body language, inflection of voice, and eye contact tell the intuitive practitioner much about an individual's health. The ability to maintain "skin" must be protected in a future high-tech world. Technology is not a master intelligence replacing human abilities. Just as a stethoscope is a tool to enhance practice, technology is only a tool.

THE FUTURE HEALTHCARE RECORD

The National Health Service in the United Kingdom is developing a global electronic patient record system that stores and distributes information between doctor and patient anywhere in the world. In the future, massive electronic data banks for healthcare information will contain cradle-to-grave information on every person. No longer will a person's health history be piecemeal, residing in the various institutions in which care was given. Instead, it will be a continuous record attached to the individual and accessible from any location in the world. When this idea becomes a reality, the **electronic health record** will reflect the current health status and lifetime medical history of an individual. Healthcare professionals will utilize information technology to capture, manage, archive, and deliver medical records anywhere in the world.

To create a global electronic patient record system, a unique patient identifier must be established. As a result of the search for a method to uniquely identify everyone in the world, the biometrics industry has flourished. **Biometrics** includes identification methods such as the fingerprint and voiceprint, as well as retinal, iris, and facial imaging. The technology records indelible characteristics that are unique to individuals—their voices, eyes, and hands—for identification. Fingerprint imaging is used in a few hospitals in the United States. It may be popular partly because it has a long track record of application in the military, law enforcement, and government. Retinal and iris scans are less accurate, and other biometric concepts are more expensive than fingerprint imaging.

PREPARING FOR THE FUTURE

In 1985, futurist Alvin Toffler described the impact of the information revolution on society when he said, "One has to be blind to be unaware that something extraordinary is happening to our entire way of life. The swift spread of microprocessors, biotechnology, the electronization of money, the convergence of computing and telecommunications, artificial intelligence—all such technological advances are accompanied by equally important social, demographic and political changes. . . . [T]aken together, they add up to nothing less than a mutation in our way of life" (p. 3).

The informatics-competent healthcare professional learns how to exploit new technology. An ignorant practitioner becomes its victim. Individuals who cannot program their videocassette recorder (VCR) are captive to the blinking 12:00 and cannot record their favorite programs. Those who are afraid to use an automatic teller machine (ATM) are limited by banking hours. Individuals can choose whether to become a master or a victim of technology. Technology will not go away. It is here to stay and will continue to reform healthcare delivery systems. Physicians, physician assistants, pharmacists, occupational and physical therapists, nurses, and social workers will all be affected in every aspect of their practice by the management and processing of healthcare information. An understanding of how information is managed and processed is vital for the leadership of the healthcare delivery system of the future.

Technology promises more and more information for less and less effort. However, as promises and visions for the future develop, balance between the promises of the future and faith in human judgment is essential. Wisdom and insight often come not from access to mountains of facts and information but from quiet reflection. What is held most valuable—morality, integrity, compassion, and caring—can be found only in the human spirit. While we embrace the future, we must remain loyal to unchanging humanity.

SUMMARY

Technology and computerization have moved civilization from the Industrial Age to the Information Age. Technology has affected and reshaped how individuals and groups communicate and interact. It has also affected the physical structure of our learning institutions, the methodology of teaching, and the style in which we learn. In many ways, technology has isolated individuals because it is possible to communicate around the world without ever leaving an office or home, but humanity still retains its need for physical contact ("skin"). Governments are realizing that the media have become a powerful force in shaping policy. Authoritarian governments find that controlling people through suppression of information has become increasingly difficult because of worldwide communication.

Healthcare is an information-dependent profession and is profoundly affected by technology. The healthcare professional spends more than 50 percent of his or her time gathering, sharing, analyzing, and seeking information. Automation of information enables the practitioner to access information in a more efficient, error-free manner. The data gathered about the practice of patient care and responses produced are essential for reporting outcomes, which is necessary in a managed-care environment.

The use of biotechnology will increase in the future for patient assessment, health monitoring, and establishment of a unique patient identifier. Patient identification will not be confined to the facility of the provider of an episode of care; instead, a "cradle-to-grave" record will be available anywhere in the world.

To function in the future, practitioners must be knowledgeable about the management of healthcare information through technology. Skills in accessing, managing, and critically examining information are becoming increasingly important for both employment and excellence in practice.

▶ LEARNING EXERCISES

1. Write a one- to two-page paper describing your vision of the use of technology in healthcare in the year 2030. Use your imagination.
2. Discuss how technology has changed the learning styles of both college students and younger students. How will this affect patient teaching? Wellness teaching?
3. Discuss whether technology isolates people or brings them together.
4. Ask the college librarian how technology has affected library science. Does this affect your ability to access information for your practice?
5. Discuss the dangers and promise of technology in the future of healthcare.
6. Interview an allied healthcare professional and write a one- to two-page summary of how he or she uses technology and envisions its use in his or her practice.

References

American Hospital Publishing, Inc. (1997, August 5). The 1997 *Hospitals & Health Networks* leadership survey. *Hospitals & Health Networks* [on-line serial]. Available at http://www.amhpi.com/hhn/doc16188.htm

Carlson, E., & Glasheen, L. (1998, April). MIT futurist sees 'connected' nation. *AARP Bulletin, 39*(4), 1, 12.

Kaplan, K. L. (1998, April). Healthcare at Kitty Hawk. *Healthcare Informatics,* 117–118.

Smith, S. E. (1998). Patient record key to medical searching. *Information Today, 15*(4), 12–14.

Swerdlow, J. L. (1995, October). Information revolution. *National Geographic, 188*(4), 5–11.

Toffler, A. (1985). *The adaptive organization.* New York: McGraw-Hill.

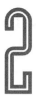

The World of Informatics

Key Words
Client
Cognitive science
Computer science
Data
Healthcare science
Informatics
Information
Information science
Knowledge

LEARNING OBJECTIVES

By the end of this chapter, you will be able to:
▶ Describe sources of information necessary for practice delivery
▶ Discuss the explosion of information
▶ Define data, information, and knowledge
▶ Describe components of informatics
▶ Define healthcare informatics

THE IMPORTANCE OF INFORMATION

The healthcare of an individual, a community, a nation, and the world is largely dependent on information. Every action taken depends on previous information and knowledge. Professional healthcare is not the same as assembly-line work. One does not go to work each day to do the same repetitive action. According to Romano, Mills, and Heller (1996, p. 2), the delivery of healthcare requires information about the:

- Science of the type of care
- Patient or client
- Provider
- Outcomes
- Process and systems for delivery of care

The "science of care" refers to the scientific basis underlying the profession that provides healthcare. Physicians have a scientific basis for their practice, as do nurses, physician assistants, occupational and physical therapists, dentists, and members of other allied health disciplines. Each profession has a unique lens through which it views the healthcare profession. Science helps determine the body of knowledge, language, and focus of that profession. Scientific rationale provides a foundation for decision making within that profession.

The patient or **client** provides the information necessary for his or her individual care. The assessment process, including both initial and ongoing assessment, consists of gathering patient information. The use of technology such as radiology and laboratory analysis assists this information-gathering process. Information is also found in the patient record, in the patient's history, and in the findings of other healthcare providers. Patient information changes and grows over time.

Information about the provider of care helps determine the type of assessment and the focus of care given. The provider of care can be an individual professional such as an occupational therapist or a psychiatrist. The provider can also be the facility in which care is provided, such as a public health department, a respiratory therapy group, or a hospital.

The outcome of treatment and care now requires more attention; historically, the process of providing care was the subject of close examination, measurement, and refinement. Before the 1990s, the Joint Commission on Accreditation of Healthcare Organizations (JCAHO) closely examined the information-gathering and decision-making processes when an organization was undergoing accreditation review. The JCAHO (1990) has revised its review to look at the "efficiency in delivery of services and for more objective evidence of the effectiveness of care" (outcome) rather than, or in addition to, the process. Although a process may be well organized and efficient, if it consistently produces a poor outcome or is ineffective, it is not a desirable process. As an example, the physician may write an order for a medication and mark the chart so that the new order demands the attention of the unit secretary. The secretary then completes the paperwork for the pharmacy and places it in a basket for review by the nurse. When the nurse notices that the order is in the basket, he or she compares it to the original order in the chart and verifies it, consults with the physician about it, or corrects the transcription of it. The nurse then puts the order in another basket for the unit secretary to send to the pharmacy *(Fig. 2.1A)*. Although everyone may understand this process, which is well organized with forms and baskets, it is time inefficient and subject to error. Automation reduces the pharmacy order process to a two-step procedure *(Fig. 2.1B)*. The order is input di-

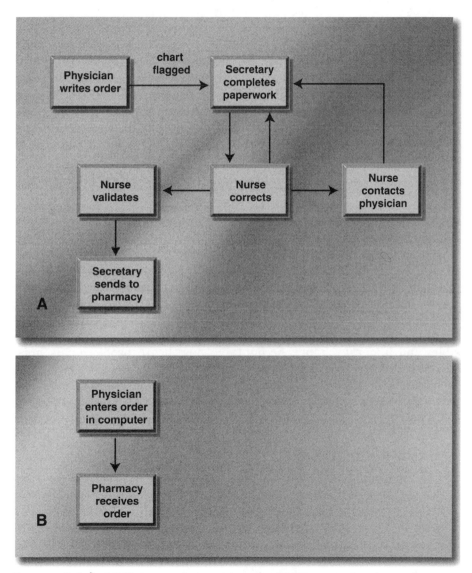

FIGURE 2.1 ▶ (*A*) Pharmacy order, manual process. (*B*) Pharmacy order, automated process.

rectly into the order entry system by the physician and is immediately read by the pharmacist. Efficiency increases and errors decline with the automated process.

Gathering and disseminating outcome information is a driving force in determining managed-care reimbursement. Managed care is discussed in more detail in Chapter 10, but in simple terms, managed-care insurance rewards physicians, facilities, and practices that produce quality outcomes in a cost-efficient manner by increasing the number of clients. However, outcomes can be difficult to measure. A reduction in medication errors can be documented with retrospective studies comparing the number of errors that occur when different processes are used. More difficult to determine are the increases in human suffering and length of hospital stay because of medication errors. The relationship between interventions and outcomes is also difficult to define and measure. How can physical therapists demonstrate that they are contributing to positive patient outcomes through their interventions in a different way from occupational therapists or nurses? When healthcare is approached holistically with interdisciplinary care, the effects of physical therapy interventions as opposed to nursing interventions on a client's functional status become difficult to distinguish.

Information about the process and systems for delivery of care assists in making decisions about the amount and type of care given. Healthcare given in an outdoor clinic in Haiti requires different interventions than care given for the same condition in a home in Europe. In America, providing care for a homeless person with diabetes differs markedly from providing care for a middle-class, otherwise healthy person with diabetes.

Information about each of these areas affects the type and amount of care given. Therefore, the information must be accurate, timely, accessible, and understandable. Accountable healthcare professionals must be more than passive recipients of information. They need to acquire the analytical skills to ask the right questions, to know where to seek answers, and to reach informed decisions on the basis of the available information.

INFORMATION EXPLOSION

Elliott (1994) suggests that keeping abreast of the revolutionary and evolutionary changes in medicine is extremely challenging. He poses the question: "[H]ow do we make sense of the roller-coaster ride we have embarked upon?" His answer is that "we turn to professional journals, textbooks, and the proceedings of specialty meetings to find answers." But medical information in scientific and medical journals has grown beyond a manageable level. Approximately 34,000 references from over 4000

Box 2.1   INFORMATION EXPLOSION

- Knowledge in 1950 doubled by 2000.
- Medical literature adds a new article every 26 seconds.
- Scientific articles published in 1980 had three times as many words as those published between 1910 and 1940.

Elliott, 1994.

journals are added monthly to the National Library of Medicine's MEDLINE database. These journals represent only 4 percent of the scientific journals currently published. Weiss (1986) suggests that if someone were to read every potentially important biomedical piece published in these journals, it would be necessary to read 6000 articles a day. By the year 2000, the knowledge available in 1950 has not only doubled but is found in 30 times as many publications *(Box 2.1)*. Elliott states that one new article is added to the medical literature every 20 seconds.

But the overabundance of information can actually keep an individual from finding the information needed. While drowning in information, the individual may starve for knowledge. Students often feel this way when they have stuffed themselves with information that has no relevance or meaning to them. John Lawton, a veteran reporter speaking to the American Association of Broadcast Journalists in 1995, said, "The irony of the information age is [that] it gives new respectability to the uninformed opinion." The question is "How much information is transferred to the minds of readers and is incorporated into practice or changes of behavior?" An in-depth discussion of this question appears in Chapter 3.

As the body of worldwide information explodes, knowing how to manage and process that information in order to make decisions that support practice is of monumental importance. Information technology provides a solution for managing the abundance of information and has become part of the daily professional life of all allied health disciplines. Throughout the past 3 decades, the literature in all healthcare fields has described the growing impact of technology on health and human services.

THE STRUCTURE OF INFORMATION

Whether delivered in conversation, captured in a set of handwritten notes, or stored in the memory of a computer, the same basic principles govern the structure and use of information in decision making. Words are often used interchangeably to describe information. Terms like "data," "information," and "knowledge" are commonly used to express the same idea. However, in the field of information processing, these terms have precise definitions.

Data is defined as discrete entities objectively described, without interpretation or context (Romano et al., 1996). For example, what does "110" mean? It could be a number, a piece of computer programming language, or a secret code. By itself, "110" means nothing.

Information is data processed into a structured form. Data that are interpreted, organized, structured, and given meaning are referred to as information. If it is determined that the systolic blood pressure of a 23-year-old man at 8 AM on the third day after admission is 110 mm Hg and the diastolic blood pressure is 70 mm Hg, that is useful information. When 110 is combined with other data, it takes on meaning. Information is also often structured in the form of a graph, such as a vital signs graph, or a report.

Knowledge is synthesized information derived from the interpretation of data, and it provides a logical basis for making decisions. Using knowledge is essential in making decisions as well as in making new discoveries. When the information about the patient's blood pressure is synthesized with information about the anatomy and physiology of the circulatory system, the pharmacokinetics of the medication to lower blood pressure, and the pathophysiology of plaque accumulation in blood vessels, the knowledge with which to make a decision about further care and treatment is clarified. The use of knowledge is vital in both making decisions and creating new knowledge *(Fig. 2.2)*.

In 1989 Graves and Corcoran used the correlation among data, information, and knowledge to suggest a model of nursing informatics. They stated that **informatics** is the management and processing of data into information and information into knowledge. Knowledge is then "transformed" into decisions and discoveries of new knowledge *(Fig. 2.3)*. The Graves and Corcoran model of "data to information to knowledge" is linear, always appearing to begin with data and end with acquired knowledge. But the process of synthesizing data into information to create knowledge is actually circular *(Fig. 2.4)*. Knowledge creates new questions and areas of research. To answer the questions, data are required that must be processed into information to create more knowledge. The purpose of this process is to provide the most accurate and up-to-date information with which to make decisions that guide practice. Having made a decision about giving medication to lower blood pressure based on the data collected, the practitioner must now gather more data to create information to produce the knowledge about the effectiveness of the medication so that a decision can be made about whether or not to continue that treatment.

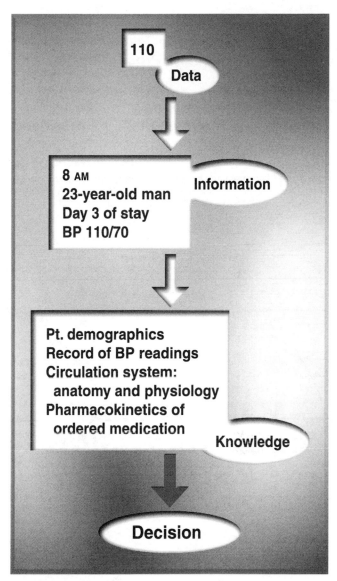

F I G U R E   2.2 ▶ Transformation of data into knowledge.

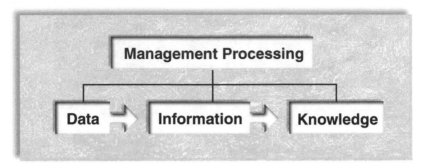

FIGURE 2.3 ▶ Conceptual framework for the study of nursing knowledge.
(Adapted from Graves, J., and Corcoran, S. [1989]. The study of nursing informatics.
Image: Journal of Nursing Scholarship, 21[4], p. 228, with permission.)

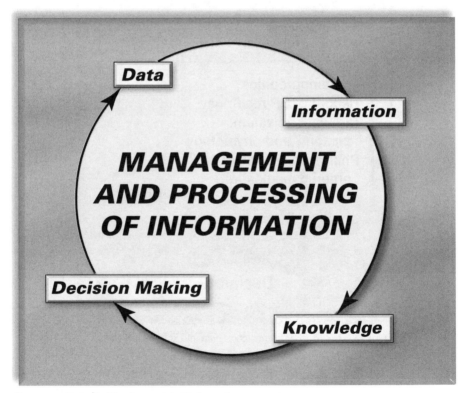

FIGURE 2.4 ▶ Circular model of information processing.

THE FIVE RIGHTS OF INFORMATION

Information has five rights:

- Right information
- Right person
- Right time
- Right place
- Right amount

To be useful, information must be the *right information*. It must be accurate, free of error, and meaningful. When examining a patient with tooth pain, a dentist does not want or need to know that the patient had braces when he was 13. The dentist wants a description of the present problem. If the pain is on the right side but the preliminary information stated that the pain was on the left side, then the information is not only incorrect, it is also misleading and potentially harmful. A real-life example brings this point home with alarming finality. In a Florida hospital, a surgeon mistakenly removed a diseased left leg instead of the more diseased right leg, as was intended (Belkin, 1997). Visual inspection could not be used to identify the leg because both legs were seriously diseased. The surgical schedule incorrectly said that the left leg was to be amputated. The error was noticed, but only one copy of the schedule was corrected. When the surgeon scrubbed for the operation, therefore, he used an operating room schedule saying that the left leg should be amputated. The wrong information had disastrous consequences.

Information must be given to the *right person* to be useful. Laboratory results that go to a unit secretary who files them are of no use. The results must be communicated to the person who will respond to them. It may be a physician, nurse, pharmacist, or therapist.

The timing of the information can be crucial to the patient's health. Information must be given at the *right time*. Laboratory results are most useful when given to the decision maker within a few minutes or hours. If the care provider does not receive the results until the patient has gone home or has had serious sequelae, the results may be useless.

Information must be delivered to the *right place*. The report of a consultation with a social worker that is misplaced in a paper chart is of no value. Laboratory results that are filed in a chart rather than communicated to the physician at his or her office or in the car or on rounds will result in delayed action and a possible increase in the number of days of illness.

Information must also come in the *right amount*. No manager wants to wade through piles of reports to retrieve one piece of information. Many reports contain much more information than anyone wants on a regular basis. Most managers want only a few pieces of information on a consistent basis. Time can be managed more efficiently and decisions made faster when only the desired information is available.

Addressing each of the five rights is important when managing information. Ignoring any of the rights weakens the usefulness of the information and can potentially harm the patient.

HEALTHCARE INFORMATICS COMPONENTS

With knowledge of the importance of information in healthcare practice and awareness of the information explosion, a need developed for specialists to manage and process information. The specialty is healthcare informatics. Informatics is multidisciplinary, and healthcare informatics *(Fig. 2.5)* is a combination of:

- Computer science
- Healthcare science
- Information science
- Cognitive science

Computer science refers primarily to the development, configuration, and architecture of computer hardware and software. The size of the memory, storage capacity, processing speed, and method by which

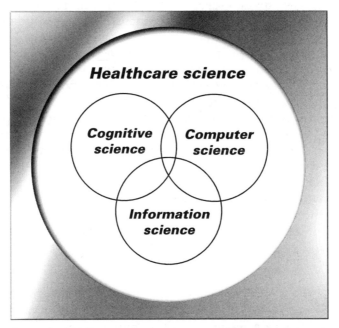

FIGURE 2.5 ▶ Components of healthcare informatics. (Adapted from Turley, J. [1996]. Toward a model for nursing informatics. *Image: Journal of Nursing Scholarship, 28*[4], p. 311, with permission.)

computers communicate are all part of computer science. The power of computer hardware doubles approximately every 18 months. "Programs" and "software" refer to the way in which a simple, logical set of instructions (algorithms) is used to solve a problem to generate a product. Algorithms help create expert systems that, along with a set of rules and laws, assist with decision making. Software develops more slowly than hardware. The development of new automated tools has radically altered the understanding of knowledge and knowledge representations.

Healthcare science is the body of knowledge on which the healthcare profession bases its practice. The sciences of anatomy, physiology, and biology, as well as the discrete knowledge that makes each profession distinctive, offer a basis for allied health professions.

Information science and information technology involve the process of sending and receiving messages. Acquiring, transmitting, processing, and perceiving information all contribute to the effectiveness of the information. Various methods communicate information: verbal, visual but nonverbal, written, and digitized. The focus of information technology is application of information tools for the solution of business problems. Information science is interested in the flow and structure of information.

Cognitive science focuses on understanding the functions of the mind. The processes of human thinking, understanding, and remembering are part of this science. It is concerned with the nature of knowledge, its components, its sources, its development, and its deployment (Gardner, 1985). How "user friendly" a computer program or piece of equipment is or how automation can reduce human error is the focus of study in cognitive science.

Turley (1996) wrote about nursing informatics, but his observations can apply to all healthcare disciplines' use of informatics. He suggested that informatics has evolved to include three special interest levels: technology, concepts, and function. He described early definitions of nursing informatics that focus on technology; he also described the use of hardware, software, and system architecture in managing and processing information. Some later informaticists (Ryan & Nagle, 1994) became interested mainly in the underlying concepts of theory, arguing that without a well-articulated theoretical basis to guide the gathering of data, the practitioner will be inundated with meaningless data and information. They stressed the need for definitions, a standardized language, and criteria for organization of the data. Other informaticists (Brennan, 1989; Schlehofer, 1992) interested in function focused on how the management and processing of information help nurses enter, organize, or retrieve information. They emphasized the usability of the applications to achieve specific purposes.

Informatics includes all these areas, but the field has become so large that it is difficult for one person to be knowledgeable in all areas. This textbook gives an overview of all of the areas of informatics.

INFORMATICS DEFINITION

Nursing and medicine are the leaders in healthcare concerning the study and application of informatics to practice, but all healthcare disciplines are realizing the need to manage and process the vast amounts of information needed to guide their practices. The term "medical informatics," coined in the mid-1970s, borrows from the French expression *informatique médicale*. It describes "those collected informational technologies which concern themselves with the patient care, medical, decision-making process" (Greenburg, 1975). Mandil (1989) uses the term "health informatics," which he defines as the use of information technology with information management concepts and methods to support the delivery of healthcare. Mandil's definition encompasses medical, nursing, dental, and pharmacy informatics, as well as all other healthcare disciplines. His definition of health informatics focuses attention on the recipient of care rather than on the discipline of the caregiver.

Each allied health discipline has distinct, discrete information needs based on the scientific basis and practice of that profession. Accordingly, each discipline has particular information requirements and may structure its information processes differently, but the basis of informatics is the same in all disciplines. The American Nurses Association (ANA) publication *The Scope of Practice for Nursing Informatics* (1994) identifies the core operations of nursing informatics as "identifying, acquiring, preserving, managing, retrieving, aggregating, analyzing, and transmitting this data, information, and knowledge to make it meaningful and useful to nurses" (p. 6). The *American Nurses Credentialing Center Catalog* (1994) states that nursing informatics practice "encompasses the full range of activities that focus on the methods and technologies of information handling in nursing. It includes the development, support, and evaluation of applications, tools, processes and structures which assist the practice of nurses with the management of data in direct care of patients."

In the broadest sense, informatics for healthcare professionals is the management and processing of information to support decision making in practice. It encompasses all information needs related to a healthcare practice. Information systems do not have to be electronic, but electronic systems certainly increase accessibility, accuracy, and efficiency. Informatics supports all areas of practice, including education, administration, and research; it also facilitates and guides the management of data.

GOAL OF INFORMATICS

The goal of informatics is to:

- Inform healthcare providers
- Expand knowledge
- Deliver efficient, well-managed care or services

The study of informatics improves the effectiveness of data assimilation, interpretation, and representation so that healthcare professionals can make informed decisions. It is no longer an elective that is "nice to know" but a necessity in today's competitive and rapidly changing healthcare delivery system.

FUTURE OF INFORMATICS

Healthcare organizations from acute care to outpatient care to home care are automating. These organizations need knowledgeable practitioners to investigate, implement, and use automation to support their practice. In the future, practitioners will be hired not so much for their knowledge of skills as for their ability to handle information to make decisions that produce favorable, cost-efficient results.

SUMMARY

Healthcare professions are information dependent. Several different sources offer information to deliver care. Each source has an effect on the delivery and type of care given. The amount of information available today has grown astronomically since 1900. No single person can learn or retain all the information that is available on any given subject. Accountable practitioners must be knowledgeable about accessing, managing, and processing information; therefore, a new healthcare specialty has arisen. It is a combination of the computer, information, cognitive, and healthcare sciences. Broadly defined, informatics is the managing and processing of information to support decision making in practice. Informatics is made up of the elements of data, information, and knowledge, and is used for decision making or creating new knowledge. The continuum of data to information to knowledge is circular, as knowledge generates new questions requiring new data. Understanding informatics is a necessity in today's healthcare practice.

▶ LEARNING EXERCISES

1. Interview a healthcare professional about his or her use of automation to support practice.
2. Search a literature database or the Internet for informatics, technology, or automation in healthcare.
3. Discuss whether a patient assessment is data, information, or knowledge.
4. Discuss the impact of technology on the healthcare professional job market. Will it replace healthcare workers? Why or why not?

5. Discuss the meaning of "science of care" for your practice. How does it affect your information needs?

References

American Nurses Association. (1994). *The scope of practice for nursing informatics* (brochure). Washington, DC: American Nurses Publishing.

American nurses credentialing center catalog. (1994). Washington, DC: American Nurses Publishing.

Belkin, L. (1997, June 15). How can we save the next victim? *The New York Times Magazine, 29*–33, 44, 50, 63, 70.

Brennan, P. (1989). Keep the nurse in nursing informatics! A comment on guidelines for reporting innovations in computer-based informatics systems for nursing. *Computers in Nursing, 7*(5), 239–240.

Elliott, S. (1994). Information overload and medical progress: When is enough too much? *Minimally Invasive Surgical Nursing, 8*(1), 23–27.

Gardner, H. (1985). *The mind's new science: A history of the cognitive revolution.* New York: Basic Books.

Graves, J., & Corcoran, S. (1989). The study of nursing informatics. *Image: Journal of Nursing Scholarship, 21,* 227–231.

Greenburg, A. B. (1975). *Medical informatics: Science or science fiction?* Unpublished manuscript.

Joint Commission on Accreditation of Healthcare Organizations. (1990, February). The Joint Commission's agenda for change. Chicago: Author.

Mandil, S. (1989, August-September). Health informatics: New solutions to old challenges. *World Health,* 2–5.

Romano, C. A., Mills, M. E., & Heller, B. R. (1996). *Information management in nursing and health care.* Springhouse, PA: Springhouse.

Ryan, S., & Nagle, L. (1994). Nursing informatics: The unfolding of a new science. In S. Grobe & E. Pluyter-Wenting (Eds.), *Nursing informatics: An international overview for nursing in a technological era.* New York: Elsevier.

Schlehofer, G. (1992). Informatics: Managing clinical operations data. *Nursing Management, 23*(7), 36–38.

Turley, J. P. (1996). Toward a model for nursing informatics. *Image: Journal of Nursing Scholarship, 28*(4), 309–313.

Weiss, P. (1986). *Health and biomedical information in Europe.* Copenhagen: World Health Organization.

3

The Right Information

LEARNING OBJECTIVES

By the end of this chapter, you will be able to:
▶ Define evidence-based practice
▶ Compare the classical model of clinical decision making with the new model

▶ Articulate the need for standards of practice
▶ Identify healthcare literature databases
▶ Discuss strategies to increase accessibility and usability of healthcare information
▶ List the items on the good practice checklist
▶ Discuss future uses of interdisciplinary information sharing

THE PROCESS OF DECISION MAKING

"Science and technology revolutionize our lives," wrote the historian Arthur M. Schlesinger Jr., "but memory, tradition and myth frame our response" (Schlesinger, 1986, p. 20). According to Millenson (1997), medicine's strongest memories, traditions, and myths revolve around the belief that a well-trained physician or health professional instinctively knows the right thing to do and will do it if given the necessary freedom and resources. He states further that there has been little effort to examine systematically the most effective treatments, to apply scientific findings consistently to patient care, or to hold practitioners accountable for improving care (p. 352). In discussing the decision-making process for patient care, Samuel Thier (1991), then president of the National Academy of Sciences Institute of Medicine, acknowledged, "Defining what does and does not work in medicine is a professional responsibility of the highest order" (p. 54). Thier concluded, however, that physicians have resisted accepting responsibility for investigating treatment outcomes.

Several positive forces are currently affecting changes in the decision-making practices of healthcare practitioners: accessibility of research and healthcare data, publicity about the human cost of medical errors, and the need to reduce the soaring cost of healthcare in the United States. Accessing the right information for clinical decision making by using the best available evidence is an important step in providing effective, quality care. Transforming new, research-based knowledge into practice is a constant challenge for all healthcare professionals. A study initially conducted in the 1930s, but still relevant today, dramatically illustrates this challenge.

In 1934 the American Child Health Association published a report chronicling a study that involved a thousand 11-year-olds in the New York City school system (American Child Health Association, 1934). The researchers examined the children and determined that 61 percent of them had already had their tonsils removed. Area physicians examined the remaining children and determined that 45 percent of them needed a tonsillectomy. Another physician gave a second opinion concerning the remaining children, stating that 44 percent of them needed a tonsillectomy. Only 65 of the original 1000 children still had their tonsils and were not advised to have them removed. The researchers determined that the diagnosis was not based on symptoms but on individual physician treatment preferences.

The report apparently did not have much effect on reducing unnecessary tonsillectomies because in the 1950s about 50 percent of the children of insured workers had their tonsils removed. "The continuance of the practice of indiscriminate T[onsillectomies] and A[denoidectomies] is indeed an enigma," wrote Harry Bakwin (1958). According to Bakwin, the sad postscript is that not only were these procedures unnecessary but also 200 to 300 children died annually between 1950 and 1955 from complications of surgery. A review of the literature through the 1950s found no evidence to support the practice of T&A (Millenson, 1997, p. 31). Another researcher noted that the removal of tonsils and adenoids in children had become "an elaborate, institutionalized, cryptic ritual" (Lipton, 1962).

Finally, as the 1970s began, the publicity concerning unnecessary T&As began to have an impact. Physicians conceded that 50 to 80 percent of tonsillectomies were probably unnecessary, and the use of the T&A procedure began to decline (Cochrane, 1971).

Performing surgery, giving treatment, and initiating other interventions without a sound scientific basis are not unusual. The same pattern of ineffective surgeries performed without benefit of a scientific rationale is repeated with hysterectomies, open-heart surgery, and treatment for ulcers (Bunker et al., 1977). Even today, women frequently undergo electronic fetal monitoring during labor even though there is no clear evidence that it accomplishes anything other than to increase the chances that the baby will be delivered by the riskier methods of cesarean section or forceps (Millenson, 1997, p. 32).

Basing practice decisions on personal inclination rather than published evidence of efficacy is not specific to physicians. It is common practice among all healthcare disciplines. During the Crimean War in the mid-1800s, Florence Nightingale, a forerunner of modern nursing, became a heroine known as the "lady with the lamp" for her midnight walks to comfort wounded British soldiers. When she returned to England after the war, she endeavored to make sense of the high mortality rates through the use of data and statistics. Elected to the British Statistical Society in 1858, she wrote a *Proposal for Improved Statistics of Surgical Operations,* which included a plan for reporting the results of care at all British hospitals in a uniform and comparable manner. Her ideas were neither accepted nor acted on in her lifetime. Over 100 years would pass before gathering and comparing data would be used to manage patient care.

Like Florence Nightingale in the 1800s, modern health researchers, payers for healthcare, and, in increasing numbers, consumers of healthcare frequently state the need for a stronger basis of scientific evidence to create standards for healthcare practices. Although few dispute the sincerity of practitioners in trying to choose the best treatment for their patients, much care derives from tradition, previous experience, and trial and error. As seen with tonsillectomies, practice patterns vary widely and personal preference rather than verifiable evidence of efficacy may be the sole determinant of treatment. However, the desire for individual autonomy, absence of measurements, and lack of communication concerning the best practices inhibit change in decision-making behavior. **Evidence-based healthcare** is a decision-making methodology that de-emphasizes intuition, unsystematic clinical experience, and pathophysiological rationale as sufficient grounds for clinical decision making and stresses the examination of evidence from clinical research.

Evidence-Based Medicine

"Evidence-based medicine" is a term coined in the 1980s at Canada's McMaster Medical School to label a clinical learning strategy (Tsafrir & Grinberg, 1998). The logo for the Evidence-Based Medicine Informatics Project (Kilman, 1997) includes the statement:

> Evidence based health care promotes the collection, interpretation, and integration of valid, important and applicable patient-reported, clinician-observed, and research-derived evidence. The best available evidence, moderated by patient circumstances and preferences, is applied to improve the quality of clinical judgments and facilitate cost-effective health care.

Sackett and colleagues (1998) define evidence-based medicine as "the conscientious, explicit, and judicious use of current best evidence in making decisions about the care of individual patients" (p. 2). Evidence-based practice requires the integration, patient by patient, of the physician's clinical expertise and judgment with the best available, relevant external evidence (Geyman, 1998).

Practitioners are constantly faced with the task of interpreting diagnostic test results, the efficacy of interventions, the potential side effects of drug therapy, and the costs of therapy. They need to know whether the information and research used to construct **practice guidelines** is sound and whether the conclusions of research articles are valid. This analysis of the decision-making process informs the individual practices of all healthcare disciplines. Not only must accountable practitioners search for the right information on which to base decisions, but they must also use information-processing tools to access and process the information.

Old Decision-Making Process

The classic approach for decision making in healthcare (Evidence-Based Medicine Working Group, 1992) involves:

- Using personal clinical experience to solve the problem
- Reviewing one's understanding of the sciences of care (biology, pathophysiology, anatomy, psychology)

- Consulting a reference text
- Asking a local expert or coworker
- Reading a review

After the problem has been isolated, the practitioner often relies on *personal experience* and acquaintance with similar symptoms to determine a course of treatment. The development of clinical experience and instinct is a crucial and necessary part of becoming a competent practitioner; however, the interpretation of information derived from clinical experience and intuition can be misleading. Because each practitioner's experience on which the solution is based is distinctive, the course of treatment chosen will also be distinctive to that practitioner. Consequently, treatment modalities vary greatly in type, cost, and duration.

Another step in the classical problem-solving method is reviewing one's *understanding of anatomy, pathophysiology, and epidemiology.* This is often accomplished by consulting *textbooks* and *reference works.* According to the Information Seeking Behaviour of Nurses (ISBN) study of students and nurses in England (Wakeham et al., 1992), 68.3 percent of all respondents often asked nursing colleagues for information on patient or client care, and the second most often used source was ward-based information (reference material). If a textbook published or updated within the previous year is at hand, the references can be followed for the appropriate passage. However, because a textbook is only as up to date as its most recent reference, all textbooks are at least partly out of date even before they are published. Most textbooks do not qualify as scientific overviews (Oxman et al., 1993). Texts have failed to recommend drug therapy up to 10 years after the drug has been shown to be efficacious and have continued to recommend therapy up to 10 years after it has been shown to be useless (http://www.med.usf.edu/CLASS/Gene/Presentation/sld004.htm). Often facilities do not attempt to keep the most recent editions of reference materials, but continue to use old textbooks.

Local experts and colleagues are a frequent source of information, as noted in the ISBN study. Asking a colleague or consultant is highly efficient and makes the most sense when the question concerns a problem that one is unlikely to encounter again. Colleagues usually base their opinion on experiential knowledge with a lack of measurable outcomes references.

Clinical decisions are also based on *reading current literature.* Although current journals are an excellent resource, most practitioners subscribe to a limited number. Their library of journals is disorganized. With 25,000 medical journals in print, retrieval of relevant and useful information in a timely manner has become almost impossible. The health professional is fortunate to find one or two useful articles in a single journal issue (Geyman, 1998).

New Decision-Making Process

The new method of clinical decision making uses both individual clinical expertise and the best available external evidence. Neither process alone is enough. Without the classical problem-solving approach, practice risks becoming tyrannized by evidence; even excellent external evidence may be inapplicable or inappropriate for an individual patient. Without the best external evidence, practice risks rapidly become out of date, to the detriment of patients and patient care. Evidence-based practice requires that the best external evidence be integrated with individual clinical expertise. External clinical evidence can inform, but can never replace, individual clinical expertise, and it is the latter that decides whether the external evidence applies to the individual patient at all and, if so, how it should be integrated into a clinical decision. The results and methods presented in research must be critically appraised for sound principles of research design. The new decision-making process, then, is to continue with the methodologies of the classical method and:

- Define the problem precisely.
- Gather needed information including a search of recent literature.
- Select the best and most relevant studies.
- Critically appraise the evidence for validity and usefulness.
- Apply information to patient problem.
- Evaluate outcomes.

—Adapted from Sackett et al., 1998.

Evidence-based care requires a precise *definition of the patient problem* to determine the information required to resolve the problem. A description of the patient problem with a request for information concerning intervention, etiology, or therapy guides the practitioner toward relevant information. Other questions may focus on comparisons of interventions or expected outcomes of the diagnosis and intervention. Sackett and colleagues (1998) suggest using advanced searching tools and formulating a four-part question containing the problem, intervention, comparison, and outcome. An example is "In a postmenopausal woman, is hormone replacement therapy more effective than no hormone replacement therapy in reducing osteoporosis?"

Conduct an efficient search of the literature, selecting the best of the relevant studies. General textbooks lack the space to include detailed quantitative information, and therefore are not a first choice for evidence searches. Specialty texts may include this type of information but are not frequently updated. The Internet is quickly becoming a vast resource for information but is often not specific enough for setting evidence-based clinical policy or applying to individual patients. **MEDLINE** and the **Cumulative Index for Nursing and Allied Health Literature (CINAHL)**, both described later in this chapter, and specialized databases are more likely to provide current evidence-based information.

Critically appraise the information for validity and usefulness. The patients in a study should have undergone both the diagnostic test in question and the reference standard or proof that they do or do not have the target disorder (Sackett et al., 1998). The criteria should not be used to discredit studies that do not fully meet the criteria but should provide a method of determining the strength of inference associated with a clinical decision.

Apply the information to the patient problem. The evidence examined must fit the patient situation at hand. The test or intervention from a study must be available, affordable, accurate, and precise for the individual patient.

Evaluate the outcome. The proof of evidence-based healthcare lies in whether patients cared for in this fashion enjoy better health. Practitioners who keep up to date by reading the current literature critically and distinguishing strong from weak evidence are more judicious in choosing the therapy they recommend. Their diagnoses also tend to be more accurate (Evidence-Based Medicine Working Group, 1992).

Evidence-Based Practice Example

One example for consideration involves a middle-aged man who experiences a grand mal seizure that is witnessed by others. He has never had a seizure before and has no recent history of head trauma. The physical examination reveals no abnormalities. The computerized axial tomographic (CAT) scan of the head and the electroencephalogram (EEG) are both normal. The patient is understandably very concerned about his risk of seizure recurrence. Using the old paradigm, the physician tells the physician assistant (PA) to instruct the patient that the risk of recurrence is high, although that risk is not quantitated. The PA emphasizes to the patient that it is important not to drive, to take the antiseizure medicine prescribed by the doctor, and to continue to see the doctor for follow-up. The patient leaves in a state of vague trepidation about his risk of subsequent seizures.

Using the new paradigm, the PA uses the computer to access MEDLINE and conducts a literature search by entering the **Medical Subject Headings (MeSH)** terms "epilepsy," "prognosis," and "recurrence." The PA also limits the search to recent publications, human subjects, and English-language articles. Processing within these limits, the program retrieves 25 relevant articles. The PA reviews the articles and finds that one fits the circumstances for this patient. Through a subscription at the facility, the search is free of charge and takes about half an hour. The results of the search show that the patient risk of recurrence at 1 year is between 43 and 51 percent, and at 3 years the risk is between 51 and 60 percent. After a seizure-free period of 18 months, the risk of recurrence would likely be less than 20 percent (Evidence-Based Medicine Working

TABLE 3.1 ▶ **COMPARISON OF OLD AND NEW DECISION-MAKING MODELS**

Old Model	New Model
Use personal clinical experience	Continue using the old model but add:
Determine the basic mechanisms of disease and pathophysiological principles	A precise definition of the problem
Use textbooks and reference material	Gather needed information, including a literature search
Consult a local expert or colleague	Critically analyze the research methods and conclusions, selecting the best and most relevant studies
Read a review	Apply the information to the patient's problem
	Evaluate the outcome

Group, 1992). The PA conveys this information to the patient, along with a recommendation that he take his medication, follow up with his doctor, and have a review of his need for medication if he remains seizure free for 18 months. The patient leaves with a clear idea of his likely prognosis *(Table 3.1).*

Using Information to Set Standards

Evidence-based practice is especially helpful when determining practice standards and guidelines. Consider a decision-making process for determining the best practice for stage 2 decubitus ulcers in home care. Each practitioner, whether from nursing, physical therapy, occupational therapy, or medicine, has his or her own experience in treating ulcers. In fact, within each discipline, every practitioner has favorite therapies, with anecdotal stories to back up their usefulness. To determine the best practice based on measurable evidence identifying the research basis for interventions and patient teaching can be important in gaining the multidisciplinary support needed for the adoption of a standard of treatment.

The **Agency for Health Care Policy and Research (AHCPR)** is a branch of the National Institutes of Health (NIH) whose mission is "to promote research designed to improve the quality of healthcare, reduce its cost, and broaden access to essential services. AHCPR's broad programs of research bring practical, science-based information to medical practitioners and to consumers and other healthcare purchasers" (AHCPR, 1998).

Established by Congress in 1989, AHCPR also provides information to healthcare consumers to help people ask the right questions and thus make more informed decisions about healthcare services (Buerhaus, 1998). In an effort to provide information to the White House's healthcare reform task-force committees in the mid-1990s, AHCPR developed practice guidelines. The guidelines are a product of interdisciplinary panels and are based on thousands of articles. According to the AHCPR home page (http://www.ahcpr.gov:80/clinic/assess.htm), the clinical guidelines provided are "based on comprehensive reviews and rigorous analyses of relevant scientific evidence. Evidence reports provide the scientific foundation for public and private organizations to use in developing tools for improving the quality of health care." Developing clinical practice guidelines in collaboration with other healthcare providers promotes interdisciplinary care, which increases the effectiveness and quality of patient care.

Research funded by AHCPR identifies gaps in knowledge about the effectiveness of treatments for prevalent, costly conditions and translates the findings of that research into useful tools for everyday clinical practice. Outcomes research prompted formation of Patient Outcomes Research Teams (PORTS), which are large, multisite, multidisciplinary projects, smaller-scale studies, and pharmaceutical outcomes studies. These projects provide the basic building blocks of the evidence for improved clinical practice and, in many cases, also include the development of tools for everyday practice (Eisenberg, 1998). As an example of the use of practice guidelines, one AHCPR-funded study reveals that the antibiotic erythromycin, used for treating community-acquired pneumonia in most outpatients aged 60 or younger, costs two-thirds less than other antibiotics and has no adverse effect on medical outcomes (Gleason et al., 1997).

Transforming Information into Practice

The need to reduce variability in practice, control costs, and improve patient care outcomes has stimulated the development of clinical paths and practice guidelines. However, systematic reviews have shown that the mere existence of these guidelines does not necessarily lead to changes in practice. Problems with the dissemination of guidelines are frequently cited as a major reason for failure to affect practice (Zielstorff, 1998). "Certainly, if clinicians are unaware of the best practices, they cannot implement them; and if they haven't been convinced of their utility, they will not use them. Even before the 'guidelines movement' came into being, nursing literature reflected a long-standing concern with the difficulties of promoting the utilization of research findings in practice" (Zielstorff, 1998).

Dissemination of new knowledge is a long-standing dilemma. Practitioners try to keep abreast of new developments through journals, conferences, and continuing education, but the information is too varied and copious for any individual to assimilate. It is becoming increasingly apparent that the major problem in practicing evidence-based healthcare is finding relevant evidence in a timely way so that it can be integrated into clinical decision making at the point of care. Implementing new information-gathering methods into common practice is imperative. As an increasing number of electronic databases become more complete and user friendly, this problem will be alleviated. The **transformation of data into knowledge** is the basis for the dissemination of information. Cognitive processing, coupled with experiences and associations, completes the knowledge transformation.

Computerization of information is not necessary to manage and process it, but automation is certainly helpful. Automated forms of healthcare information include the electronic health record, **literature databases**, e-mail, online journals, electronic bulletin boards, the Internet, the intranet, and Compact Disk–Read-Only Memory (CD-ROM) publications.

LITERATURE DATABASES

Automated literature databases provide access to relevant literature and are an important research source in all disciplines. These databases offer speed, flexibility, currency, and convenience in retrieving relevant healthcare information. A database usually covers a specific list of periodicals or other publications that give the database defined boundaries. Databases are generally specific to one field such as healthcare, social sciences, education, mathematics, or nuclear science. The list of journals covered in a database determines and assures the level of quality of its contents. The database may be limited to research journals or may include trade magazines as well. All editorial decisions made about the content of the database will affect the nature of its content. Databases provide a defined, controlled, predictable, and efficient means of finding relevant information on a particular topic.

A vast array of specialized healthcare databases is available *(Table 3.2)*. Databases are produced by the government, by nonprofit private organizations, and by for-profit private companies. With a personal computer and a modem, a subscriber can access a distant vendor such as BRS Information Technologies, PaperChase, the National Library of Medicine (NLM), and DIALOG Information Services. All offer user-friendly programs for nonlibrarians. Institutions, library subscriptions, or direct contact with a vendor can provide access to databases. Some databases, such as MEDLINE, are free. For other databases the user, either an individual or an institution, must pay an hourly use rate, a fee to print citations, and telecommunications fees. CD-ROM services can also be purchased from vendors. This generally includes a CD-ROM version of the database sent to an individual subscriber and replaced quarterly or annually. Special rates are often offered to students. Subscriptions to databases vary from $50 to $1000 per year.

TABLE 3.2 ▶ SELECTED DATABASES

Database	Description
AIDS Cancer	An index of cancer and AIDS research gathered from worldwide scientific literature, as summarized in *Virology & AIDS Abstracts, Oncogenes and Growth Factors Abstracts,* and *Immunology Abstracts.*
Article 1st	Contains journal articles in science, technology, medicine, social science, business, the humanities, and popular culture.
CINAHL	Covers nursing, allied health, biomedical, and consumer health journal articles, as well as publications of the American Nurses Association and the National League for Nursing.
FactSearch	Guide to statistical statements on current social, economic, political, environmental, and health issues derived from newspapers, periodicals, newsletters, and documents such as the *Christian Science Monitor,* the *Congressional Record,* congressional hearings, *Daily Press Briefings* of the White House, the U.S. State Department and U.S. Department of Defense, and Australian, British, and Canadian *Parliamentary Debates.* Web links to free full text are frequently included.
Health Reference Center (HRCtr)	A multisource database for health and wellness research. Rich with full text documents, it draws from medical and consumer periodicals, health newsletters, reference books, referral books, referral information, topical overviews, and pamphlets. Designed especially for lay research, HRCtr provides information in terms that the nonmedical professional can understand. It includes indexes for 165 medical journals and consumer health magazines, with full text for more than 110 of these titles; full text of health-related articles from more than 1500 general-interest periodicals; full text of 6 medical reference books; more than 1800 medical topic overviews from Clinical Reference Systems; and contact information for support groups, hotlines, and research centers from the *Complete Directory for People with Chronic Illness.*
MEDLINE	Lists articles from journals published internationally, covering all areas of biomedicine.
PsycINFO	Lists articles from journals on psychology and related fields.

Each entry in the database contains an article citation, subject headings describing the article, and a text summary of the article called an "abstract." Other information about the article may also be included, such as the name of the author(s), the name of the institution at which the research was done, and the language in which the article was published. CINAHL, PubMed, and MEDLINE are the most frequently used healthcare databases.

CINAHL covers nursing, allied health, biomedical, and consumer health journals, as well as publications of the American Nurses Association and the National League for Nursing (NLN). This database also includes relevant articles culled from the educational, behavioral science, business, information science, and popular literature arenas. The database offers more than 900 periodicals, including articles from 1982, with most articles from 1986 to the present containing an abstract. Updating occurs monthly. The coverage of nursing journals is approximately the same as that of MEDLINE; however, the subject heading lists, features, and content are more specific to nursing.

The National Library of Medicine produces MEDLINE, which is considered the premier biomedical database, with over 3800 publications, including over 300 nursing titles. The database includes all areas of biomedical publications since 1966 and is international in scope. Numerous other databases are available through private organizations, government agencies, and library services.

SEARCHING THE LITERATURE

In a database, the information about each article is divided into numerous fields *(Box 3.1)*. The major fields consist of the author, the article title, the source (journal publication information), the descriptors (medical subject or MeSH headings, see below), and the abstract (when available). Because each document is divided into these major fields of information,

---

Box 3.1   EXAMPLE OF DATABASE FIELDS

UNIQUE IDENTIFIER
89183682

AUTHORS
Poole A.

TITLE
Taken to Task [Interview by Jane Feinmann]

SOURCE
Nursing Times. 85(10):19, 1989 Mar 8–14.

NLM JOURNAL CODE
O9u

COUNTRY OF PUBLICATION
England

MeSH SUBJECT HEADINGS
Great Britain
Human
*nursing services/og [Organization & Administration]
Societies, Nursing
State Medicine/og [Organization & Administration]

the searcher has several options in retrieving and limiting a list of documents on a particular topic: (1) searching by author, (2) searching by subject, (3) searching by year(s), or (4) searching by source.

Every database uses a specific language for indexing subject headings that can be identified by becoming familiar with the thesaurus in the database. MEDLINE uses Medical Subject Headings (MeSH) and Medical Subject Headings: Tree Structures. CINAHL uses a Subject Heading List and lists the topics in alphabetical order. Finding the keywords used by that database to index the content improves searching effectiveness. The first and most important step in a literature search is identifying the question for which the searcher wants an answer. Using broad terms such as "malaria," "aging," or "community health" results in thousands of possible articles. Narrowing the search to "malaria treatment," "aging demographics," or "community wellness programs" reduces the amount of material to review. Limiting the search to a specific time frame (1995–1999) or to a language (English) focuses the search on the most relevant information. The success of a search is determined by how specifically the searcher can describe the subject. CINAHL is generally more user friendly for the novice searcher because of its use of allied health subject headings. MEDLINE, which is free through the NIH, continues to be the authority for comprehensive coverage of the international biomedical field and is slightly more current. When a searcher requires extensive coverage of a subject area, he or she can consult both databases to ensure that all relevant citations are found.

WHAT IS THE PROBLEM?

If evidence-based practice produces the most desired patient outcomes and the evidence is accessible through the most current research in literature databases, why isn't the information used to guide and set standards of practice? Why are most practitioners still relying on the old method of decision making? The results of the Establishing the Value of Information to Nursing Continuing Education (EVINCE) study in England (Urquhart & Davies, 1997) demonstrates that nurses, midwives, and health visitors highly value information that benefits their practices, but according to Bohannan and LeVeau (1986), health professionals underuse their professional literature. Studies reveal that nurses use hospital libraries less often than other professionals and rarely subscribe to journals (Blythe et al., 1995). In daily nursing practice, information resources that could improve decision making about client care are also underused. Few practitioners use the opportunities provided by information technology to access professional literature as a tool for applying new research to their practice. Barriers to evidence-based practice include lack of prioritizing evidence-based behavior, time, access, education, and modeling *(Box 3.2)*.

BOX 3.2   BARRIERS TO EVIDENCE-BASED PRACTICE

- Failure to prioritize evidence-based behavior
- Lack of time
- No education
- No role modeling

Decision Making Not Valued

Dealey and Berker (1986) report that decision-making ability is not always a significant priority in healthcare. Their study indicates that the ideology of nursing emphasizes practical rather than intellectual knowledge, inhibiting information seeking.

Lack of Access

Lack of convenient access to literature resources is also a barrier to evidence-based practice. Hospitals usually have library facilities, but they are physically removed from patient care areas and may not be open 24 hours a day or available to all professionals. Some libraries are restricted to the medical staff, may be locked after business hours, and therefore are not even accessible. Individual clinics, outpatient facilities, and ambulatory care sites seldom have library services. Accessing information is very time consuming when a trip to another facility, perhaps even in another community, is necessary.

Lack of Education

Even when library resources are readily available, many healthcare professionals do not have the education to use the technology to access and retrieve information relevant to clinical decision making. Computer education is now common in colleges and universities, but many experienced practitioners are not computer literate. In a work environment, training in the use of hardware and software does not always accompany its installation, or the training can be minimal.

Lack of Information-Seeking Modeling

Professionals have few evidence-based practice colleagues who take the time to add critical appraisal of the evidence-based healthcare process to decision making about individual patient problems. The classic method for decision making is generally accepted for practice and is the modeled behavior. A generation of professionals following the new method of decision making is necessary before the behavior can be modeled for the novice.

EXAMPLE OF UNIT-BASED LITERATURE SEARCH ACCESS

In the early 1990s, Royle and colleagues (1995) conducted a study on a 32-bed medical and hematology unit in a Canadian hospital to assess whether nurses would use a literature research and retrieval system if it were made available in the workplace and if the nurses received training in its use. Researchers believed that electronic access to information on the unit would encourage nurses to incorporate literature use into their practice (Royle et al., 1995). The researchers equipped the nursing unit with a personal computer with a CD-ROM drive. The nurses had access to six databases and the Health Science Library's online catalog. In addition, they received user manuals, search aids, textbooks, and reference books on medical-surgical and oncology nursing. The nurses also received extensive training in the use of the hardware and software, the mechanics of a literature search, and the techniques of article analysis.

The actual use of the system by nurses was measured over a 6-month period and involved 29 staff nurses who attempted almost 200 searches. CINAHL and MEDLINE were the most frequently used databases. "Before the information system was implemented, nurses had been unaware of the scope of their professional literature and read little research material. After the study, they were much more aware of materials available to them and how to access them. They were reading more research abstracts and articles and reported that using articles and texts in educational projects helped them appreciate the variety of opinions held on health science topics. The nurses also claimed that having access to literature about clinical issues gave them confidence in dealing with patients and other health professionals and allowed them to contribute more fully to the multidisciplinary health care team" (Blythe et al., 1995, p. 344). After the study, the nurses agreed that finding uninterrupted time to use the system was still a problem. Without the system on the unit, they doubted that they would have the time to visit the library and retrieve articles. They also identified the lack of value given information-seeking behavior in their job design and work expectations. Despite problems in using the literature search and retrieval system, the nurses retained their enthusiasm and wanted to continue searching the literature after the project ended.

STANDARDS OF INFORMATION SEEKING

Funded by the British Library Research and Development Department, the EVINCE research project in 1996 sought to establish how nurses, midwives, and health visitors used information. The study focused on the value of information to these nursing professionals for their present and future competence (Urquhart & Davies, 1997). The project resulted in a **good practice checklist** for library access *(Box 3.3)*.

Box 3.3   Good Practice Checklist

1. Every nurse should have access to a free library service,
   funded by his or her employer, that contains appropriate
   literature and multimedia resources.
2. Library services should have flexible operating hours and be
   staffed by qualified librarians.
3. Nurses should have equal rights, similar to those of other
   healthcare professionals, to paid study time to update their
   practice.
4. Every nurse should have access to and training on the
   Internet and appropriate databases, including Cochrane and
   The Centre for Reviews and Dissemination (a source of
   systematic reviews of the literature).
5. Every nurse should be educated in systems and services to
   support evidence-based practice.

Source: Urquhart, C., & Davies, R. (1997). The impact of information. *Nursing Standard, 12*(8),
28–31. London: RCN Publishing Co., with permission.

The checklist targets nurses, but the same information needs and
principles for sound practice apply to all healthcare professionals. Members of all healthcare professions have a responsibility to work with representative professional organizations, other healthcare providers, and
healthcare facilities to (1) understand the importance of evidence-based
care to optimal patient outcomes, (2) overcome the barriers to evidence-based practice, and (3) provide the information-seeking tools necessary
to search the literature.

FUTURE CONSIDERATIONS

Collaborative information seeking, sharing, and retrieving among all
healthcare practitioners has become a daily occurrence, and indications
are that information-seeking behavior will increase in importance as
practitioners increasingly receive calls to work interprofessionally. Computers and related technologies will become a vital tool, allowing members of these teams to communicate with each other concerning individual patient care and planning. Software companies are beginning to
develop evidence-based treatment protocols that are constantly updated
with current research and outcome studies. In the near future, expert
systems, perhaps tied to centralized databases reflecting relative success
with specific populations and problems, may be an online requirement.
Practitioners will access empirical data referencing appropriate treatment protocols, and the determination of effectiveness will be based on
standardized measures related to treatment goals. Computer-generated

optimal protocols of care developed by recognized experts will guide treatment decisions.

In the future, patients may respond routinely by computer to a standardized set of questions about their problems before their appointment with a healthcare professional. These data will be available to both the patient and the healthcare team for baseline information and for tracking progress toward a treatment goal according to the interventions of the protocol. Analysis of the data gathered from a cross section of patients with similar diagnoses will determine future protocols.

SUMMARY

An empirical, evidence-based practice model of decision making will ground patient care, providing standards by which outcomes of care can be measured and evaluated. However, multiple barriers still prevent widespread use of evidence-based practice. Healthcare professionals in all disciplines must work to overcome these barriers so that information-seeking behavior becomes a valued component of the healthcare delivery system.

▶ LEARNING EXERCISES

1. Examine the information resources available at a clinical facility. Assess both computerized and hard-copy resources. Determine their accessibility, currency, relevance, usage, and ease of use.
2. Formulate a healthcare question concerning either a patient care or personal health/illness issue. Look for answers to the question on several databases. Compare the ease of use, helpfulness in answering the question, and amount of time necessary to find the answer.
3. Discuss the decision-making process with a healthcare practitioner. Does he or she use the old paradigm or the new paradigm?
4. Identify the difference between a journal database and a database for books.

References

Agency for Health Care Policy and Research. (1998). Web site. http://www.ahcpr.gov/about/about.htm

American Child Health Association. (1934). *Physical defects: The pathway to correction*. New York: Author.

Bakwin, H. (1958, March). The tonsil-adenoidectomy dilemma. *Journal of Pediatrics, 52*(3), 339–361.

Blythe, J., Royle, J. A., Oolup, P., Potvin, C., & Smith, S. D. (1995). Linking the professional literature to nursing practice: Challenges and opportunities. *American Association of Occupational Health Nurses, 43*(6), 342–345.

Bohannan, R. W., & LeVeau, B. F. (1986). Clinicians' use of research findings: A review of the literature with implications for physical therapists. *Physical Therapy, 66,* 40–45.

Buerhaus, P. I. (1998). Nursing's first senior scholar at the U.S. Agency for Health Care Policy and Research. *Image: Journal of Nursing Scholarship, 30*(4), 311–314.

Bunker, J. P., Barnes, B. A., & Mosteller, F. (Eds.). (1977). *Costs, risks and benefits of surgery.* New York: Oxford University Press.

Centre for Evidence Based Medicine. 1997. NHS Research and Development (producer and distributor). Web site http://cebm.jr2.ox.ac.uk/

Cochrane, A. L. (1971). *Effectiveness and efficiency: Random reflections on health services.* London: Nuffield Provincial Hospitals Trust.

Dealey, C. L., & Berker, M. (1986). Action speaks louder than words. *Nursing Times, 82*(29), 37–39.

Eisenberg, J. (1998). Federal scene: Agency for health care policy and research. *Annual Epidemiology, 5*(8), 283–285.

Evidence-Based Medicine Working Group. (1992, November 4). Evidence-based medicine. *Journal of the American Medical Association, 268*(17), 2420–2425.

Geyman, J. P. (1998). Evidence-based medicine in primary care: An overview. *Journal of the American Board of Family Practitioners, 11*(1), 46–56.

Gleason, P. P., Kapoor, W. N., Stone, R. A., Lave, J. R., Obrosky, D. S., Schulz, R., Singer, D. E., Coley, C. M., Marrie, T. J., & Fine, M. J. (1997). Medical outcomes and antimicrobial costs with the use of American Thoracic Society guidelines for outpatients with community-acquired pneumonia. *Journal of the American Medical Association, 278*(1), 32–39.

Kilman, Y. (1997). Evidence-based medicine (online). Web site http://www.med.usf.edu/CLASS/Gene/ebm.htm

Lipton, S. D. (1962). On psychology of childhood tonsillectomy. In R. S. Eissler (Ed.), *Psychoanalytic study of the child* (pp. 363–417). New York: International Universities Press.

Millenson, M. L. (1997). *Demanding medical excellence.* Chicago and London: University of Chicago Press.

Oxman, A. D., Sackett, D. L., & Guyatt, G. H. (1993). Users' guide to the medical literature. *Journal of the American Medical Association, 270*(17), 2093–2095.

Royle, J. A., Blythe, J., Potvin, C., Oolup, P., & Chan, I. M. (1995). Literature search and retrieval system in the workplace. *Computers in Nursing, 13*(1), 25–31.

Sackett, D. L., Richardson, W. S., Rosenberg, W., & Haynes, R. B. (1998). *Evidence-based medicine: How to practice and teach EBM* (7th ed.). London: Churchill Livingstone.

Schlesinger, A. M. (1986, July 27). The challenge of change. *New York Times,* 20–21.

Thier, S. O. (1991, July 1). Health care reform: Who will lead? *Annals of Internal Medicine, 115*(1), 54–58.

Tsafrir, J., & Grinberg, M. (1998, January). Who needs evidence-based healthcare? *Bulletin of the Medical Library Association, 41.*

Urquhart, C., & Davies, R. (1997). The impact of information. *Nursing Standard, 12*(8), 28–31.

Wakeham, M., Houghton, J., & Beard, S. (1992). *The information seeking behaviour of nurses.* Boston Spa, Wetherby: British Library Document Supply Centre.

Zielstorff, R. D. (1998, May/June). Online practice guidelines: Issues, obstacles, and future prospects. *Journal of the American Medical Informatics Association, 5*(3), 227–236.

4

The Human Side of Information

LEARNING OBJECTIVES

By the end of this chapter, you will be able to:
▶ Define human factors
▶ Discuss the importance of human factors in device design
▶ List the attributes of usability
▶ Describe the human capabilities that are important in human factors design
▶ Apply the analysis and design phases in human factors engineering
▶ Discuss types and causes of human error
▶ List suggestions for reducing design errors

In 1986, Voyne Ray Cox was a patient in the East Texas Cancer Center of Tyler, Texas. Ray, as he was commonly called, had surgery to remove a tumor from his left shoulder and was receiving follow-up radiation treatments. He had every reason to believe that between the surgery and the radiation treatments he would overcome his cancer and return to his work in the oil fields. His first eight radiation treatments had gone well, and he did not believe that the ninth session would cause him any problems.

The cancer center had state-of-the-art radiation equipment. The Therac-25 was a million-dollar piece of equipment capable of delivering a beam of high-energy radiation to any point on or in the human body. The key to successful radiation treatment was twofold: hitting the cancer cells with pinpoint accuracy and administering many separate treatments involving relatively low doses rather than a single treatment with one large dose. Ray was receiving the small doses; his schedule called for many more sessions in the treatment room.

The technician was very familiar with the Digital Equipment Corporation VT100 terminal connected to a PDP-11 computer to control the radiation. Using the control system, the technician could aim the accelerator with pinpoint accuracy and fire a direct radiation beam of the prescribed intensity at the site. Ray should not have felt a thing.

However, the video camera did not function in the technician control room on the day of Ray's ninth radiation treatment because it was not plugged in. The voice intercom between the two rooms was also inoperative. But neither the technician nor Ray seemed concerned about these communication devices because all previous treatments had taken place without incident.

According to Casey (1993), the Therac-25 had two modes of operation. A high-powered x-ray mode utilized the full 25 million electron volt capacity of the machine. "It was selected by typing an 'x' on the keyboard. This put the machine on maximum power and automatically inserted a thick metal plate just beneath the beam. When passed through the metal plate, the beam transformed into an x-ray, which [ir]radiate[d] tumors inside the body. The plate also lowered the intensity of the beam" (p. 15). The other setting lowered the power mode selected by pressing "e" on the keyboard. Ray was scheduled to receive the second option: a painless, low dose of about 200 rads to the spot on his shoulder.

After the technician carefully positioned Ray on the metal treatment table, she entered the control room to begin the treatment. She typed in "x" and immediately realized that she had entered the wrong mode. She had intended to enter an "e" for the lower dose setting but had entered "x," the higher x-ray setting. Because the treatment had not begun, the technician corrected her error by following the guidelines established by Therac's manufacturer. She used the "up" key to select the edit functions and corrected the electron beam setting. The screen display verified that she now had the correct setting. She had corrected her initial error within 8 seconds.

Unfortunately, the designers of the Therac-25, Atomic Energy of Canada, Ltd. (AECL), had never considered the possibility of that sequence of keystrokes occurring in that short a segment of time. In the thousands of treatments already delivered by the Therac-25 machine, this sequence of inputs had never occurred; therefore, it had never been tested. Instead of responding as expected and correcting the input error, the machine retracted the metal barrier plate for the x-ray mode but proceeded to deliver a full 25,000 rads to Ray's shoulder when the technician pressed the beam key. This was equivalent to 25 million electron volts.

Ray saw a flash of blue light, heard a frying sound, and felt an excruciating pain like a hot poker in his back. He rolled to his side, feeling that his shoulder was on fire. Inside the control room, the technician was unaware of Ray's plight because the communication with the treatment room was not functioning. Her computer screen did light up with a malfunction message indicating that the machine was not functioning and that treatment had *not* been initiated. The technician quickly reset the machine and fired it again. The second flash of blue light and the radiation blast caught Ray in the neck. The pain was more intense than anything he had ever endured. He tried to call out, but the technician could not hear him. The machine still displayed an error message. A third beam of radiation hit Ray before he rolled off of the table and fled the room.

On examination, no physical injury of Ray was apparent, and no malfunction was apparent in the machine. The hospital continued to use the machine that day because other patients were waiting for their treatments. Three weeks later, the same sequence of events produced a blue light and extreme pain in another patient. This time the AECL and other users of the Therac-25 were alerted to the problem. Subsequent investigation found similar overdoses in clinics in Marietta, Georgia; Ontario, Canada; and Yakima, Washington. Four months later, Ray died of massive radiation poisoning (Casey, 1993, p. 19).

DEFINITION OF HUMAN FACTORS ENGINEERING

Human errors account for a growing amount of death and misfortune in the skies, waterways, workplaces, and hospitals. "Structurally sound aircraft plummet to the earth, ships run aground in calm seas, industrial machines run awry, and the instruments of medical science maim and kill unsuspecting patients, all because of incompatibilities between the way things are designed and the way people perceive, think, and act" (Casey, 1993, p. 9). Because of these incompatibilities, a growing body of knowledge known as **human factors** has developed.

According to Salvendy (1987), human factors is the body of knowledge of human abilities, limitations, and characteristics that is relevant to how humans interact with their environment. It is the application of the science of psychology (human sensation, perception, cognition, and response execution) and engineering (knowledge of the design of tools, machines, systems, and jobs) for safe, comfortable, and effective human use. Human factors focuses on designing for human psychological, social, physical, and biological characteristics. The goal of human factors is to apply knowledge of human beings to the design of systems that work, accommodating the limits of human performance and exploiting the advantages of the human operator in the process (Wickens, 1992).

HISTORY OF HUMAN FACTORS

Although not known at the time as human factors engineering, the discipline may have begun in the early 1900s when Frank and Lillian Gilbreth began their work in motion study and shop management (Wickens, 1992). While studying surgical operating teams, the Gilbreths found that surgeons spent about half of their operating time searching for instruments on the surgical tray. To increase efficiency in the operating team, they instituted the procedure still used today, whereby the surgeon obtains an instrument by calling for it and extending his or her hand to a nurse, who places the instrument in the proper position for use. Despite the work of people like the Gilbreths, the idea of adapting machines for more efficient human use did not capture the imagination of manufacturers or the public and was not highly exploited at that time.

During World War II, rather than looking at the machine-human interface, the armed forces emphasized extensive training to reduce errors. However, it soon became evident that even with rigorous selection of personnel and subsequent training, errors in using complex equipment, including airplane crashes, still occurred at an alarming rate. At the end of the war in 1945, both the United States and Britain established engineering psychology laboratories, where the human factors profession was born. The terms "human factors," "human usability engineering," and "ergonomics" are often used interchangeably to describe the process used to achieve highly usable equipment. Currently, the term "human factors" is most often used in the United States and "ergonomics" is more common in Europe.

On March 28, 1979, an accident at a U.S. nuclear power plant had a major impact on the public awareness of human factors. The incident at Three Mile Island, located just outside Harrisburg, Pennsylvania, began with a simple clog in the feedwater lines of Turbine No. 1. As a result of this clog, the radioactive core failed to receive the constant cooling water that carried away the heat produced by the reactive process. The alternate feedwater system failed because the maintenance crew, who had since gone off duty, had blocked it. The automatic safeguards, however, continued to function properly. Cobalt rods descended into the core to slow down the reactive process, and a pressure relief valve opened to "bleed off" some of the high-pressure overheated vapor from the primary cooling loop. Once the temperature was reduced to normal, the automatic relief valve received a signal to close. At this point, a second error occurred: the valve did not close.

The crew tried to make sense of the multitude of lights, signals, and alarms signaling the problems. Although they were able to understand most of the information, one display was misleading. The design of the display for the pressure valve supposedly indicated what was to happen, not what actually happened. The display indicated that the valve was shut. The automated safeguards continued to operate, and an emergency pump switched on to supply the system with a now badly needed source of coolant. At that point, the supervisors made a critical decision. With instruments showing that the pressure was already high, and that the relief valve had closed, the operators decided to override the controls manually and shut off the emergency pump. The core was thereby deprived of the vital cooling water it needed, and the incident soon accelerated to the point of no return.

A detailed study of the Three Mile Island incident by Rubinstein and Mason (1979) revealed three things. First, no single fault, mistake, event, or malfunction caused the situation at Three Mile Island. Rather, responsibility was distributed across a number of sources. Second, human error was involved at several levels, from the incorrect decision to shut down the emergency coolant to the human decisions in the design of a relief valve system that told operators what the valve was commanded to do, not what it did. Third, and most important, the overwhelming complexity of the information presented to the human operators and the confusing display format were probably sufficient to guarantee that somewhere along the line, the human ability to attend, perceive, remember, decide, and act (process information) would become overloaded. The incident at Three Mile Island brought the importance of human factors to the attention of average person.

In the years since Three Mile Island, the computer revolution has propelled the discipline of human factors into the limelight. Information about ergonomically designed computer equipment, user-friendly software, and human factors is prevalent in newspaper and magazine articles dealing with computers and people. However, despite the growing expertise in human-machine interaction, disasters are not a thing of the past. Daily news reports of railway and airline crashes and the toll on human lives from medical mistakes continue as reminders of the importance of human factors design.

HUMAN OR MACHINE

According to Wickens (1992, p. 4), many human-machine systems do not work as well as possible because requirements are imposed on the human user that are incompatible with the way the user attends, perceives, thinks, remembers, decides, and responds, that is, the way in which he or she processes information. With increased technological development in the twentieth century, systems have become increasingly complex, with more and more interrelated elements, forcing the designer to consider the distribution of tasks between human and machine. For example, consider the increase in velocity with which a driver must contend, from driving the Conestoga wagon of the early pioneers migrating from the East Coast to the West Coast of the United States to the present-day operation of supersonic fighter jets. If the driver of the Conestoga wagon failed to respond to a change in function within 2 seconds, little occurred. By contrast, the failure of a 2-second response by the pilot of a speeding jet carrying nuclear weapons could be disastrous. Incompatibilities between human limitations and machine capabilities have led system designers to consider what functions to allocate to humans and what functions to allocate to machines, which in turn necessitates a close analysis of human performance in different kinds of tasks.

APPLICATION OF HUMAN FACTORS TO DESIGN

Human factors professionals study the abilities and limitations of humans in processing information as a means of determining which information is best controlled by humans and which by machines. When a device or machine is too complex or counterintuitive, its safe and efficient use can be compromised. Similar to a healthcare professional, the human factors professional applies scientific knowledge to real-world, practical situations. A healthcare practitioner initiates contact with a new client by eliciting a history of the present illness or situation that led the client to seek professional care. Likewise, a human factors professional gathers information about the end user's needs and environment to start the diagnostic inquiry. A healthcare practitioner also elicits the client's past medical history to learn about previous situations and treatments. A human factors professional looks at similar situations that have occurred with technology, both good and bad. With the healthcare practitioner, a physical examination usually follows the history and involves most body systems to fully determine the extent of the problem, which may not always be obvious to the client. The human factors professional performs tests to observe and analyze the interaction between the user and the present environment. Alternatively, the relationship between the user and a prototype of the new technology may be analyzed to reveal undisclosed problems and to re-evaluate basic design decisions. Both the healthcare practitioner and the human factors professional use an iterative or repetitive process, which allows changes in basic initial assumptions. Both set standards for determination of what is deemed to be "well" and "sick." Just as practitioners learn how to ask the right questions and how to respond with therapeutic communication, the human factors professional acquires the ability to partner with the user to design a system, machine, or program to best meet the user's needs. The resource constraints for the practitioner are just as real for human factors professionals as for healthcare professionals, prompting them to choose efficient rather than exhaustive methods.

According to Gosbee and Ritchie (1997), many medical software companies (e.g., SMS, HBOC, and Cerner) are just beginning to embrace human factors in the design of their programs. IBM and other large information systems companies have well-established human factors departments and are involved in medical software projects. Even healthcare delivery organizations and managed-care companies (e.g., the Mayo Clinic, Health Systems Technologies) have a growing appreciation of the usability of information systems. Scientific and trade societies in the medical software arena, however, are just beginning to appreciate human factors tools and to understand the role of human factors in product design.

WHY HUMAN FACTORS ARE IMPORTANT IN MEDICAL DEVICE DESIGN

Medical devices designed without thought for human factors can lead to patient injuries and even death. Not only the abilities and environments of acute-care medical personnel, but also the increasing use by laypeople of medical equipment in home settings must be considered during design. Historically, the end user of healthcare products was always the clinician responsible for providing the care to the patient. This is no longer true; the **end user** of many products is now the patient rather than the nurse, therapist, or physician. In addition, medical devices are used in a variety of settings including radiology departments, pediatric units, critical care and emergency departments, outpatient clinics, ground and air ambulances, operating rooms, and homes—all of which may require slightly different human factors engineering considerations.

Environmental factors such as noise, emergency situations requiring speed, improper cleaning, poor lighting, variable temperatures, and humidity compromise the ability to use equipment. Inadequate training, poorly written directions, fatigue, and stress also compromise performance. In addition, healthcare personnel who work in many different units or settings are constantly subjected to a variety of devices that are frequently upgraded, changed, or different from one context to another.

For devices to be used safely and effectively, the design for the interaction between user and machine must acknowledge users' capabilities, stress levels, working environments, and training needs. Studies by the Center for Devices and Radiological Health (CDRH) state that many of the causes of serious equipment errors in use are a direct result of poor equipment design and cannot be overcome by improved training of the users (Saladow, 1996). The CDRH concludes that the issues related to equipment design and human factors engineering are more important than ever in helping users learn how to use equipment effectively and correctly, especially given the increasing complexity of the technology that must be made available in certain healthcare delivery environments.

The CDRH studies demonstrate that even small, seemingly unimportant design flaws can result in significant user problems (Saladow, 1996). Identified as potential areas of concern are:

• Knobs and dials
• Device markings
• Legibility of information
• Tubings and connectors
• Software design

Because laypeople use medical products at home, the importance of human considerations becomes evident. Elderly persons are good examples of the need to consider human limitations as they struggle with diminished dexterity, reduced hearing and vision, and slowed cognitive processes. These normal changes associated with aging affect the manner in which the person interacts with common medical products and devices. As vision decreases, increased lighting and less cluttered displays on devices are necessary for easy functioning. A design issue that affects all healthcare environments is device markings that become worn or difficult to read over time and can cause errors in the use of equipment and potential accidents in the care of the patient.

Perhaps the largest area of concern as healthcare delivery spreads out over a continuum of care and struggles to become increasingly cost effective is software design. As computer software becomes more sophisticated, the ability of the manufacturer to develop sophisticated yet easy-to-understand and easy-to-use software is of critical importance. It is not unusual for a device to contain control keys that have multiple functions or require the user to depress keys in a specific order. A common example is the use of the keys "Control," "Alt," and "Delete" to reboot a personal computer. Ineffective design can lead to significant user error, potential patient harm, and the high cost of healthcare, as related in the story of Ray Cox.

HUMAN FACTORS ENGINEERING METHODS AND PROCESSES

A human factors engineer (HFE) or psychologist uses the knowledge of human capabilities and limitations, theory, and modeling for specification, design, development, testing, analysis, and evaluation of products or systems for human use (Stramler, 1993). Designing for effective human use is crucial to optimal device use. An understanding of the discipline of human factors is important for healthcare professionals involved in the management and processing of information (informatics). Knowledge of human factors increases understanding of why devices and software are hard to learn and use and enables healthcare professionals to become better consumers when selecting medical equipment or devices. An adequate understanding of human capabilities and limitations, and the application of that knowledge, are inherent in good product design. Usability has five important attributes:

- **Learnability**—Is the system easy to use so that the user can quickly accomplish work? Walt Disney's Epcot Center in Florida is full of automated kiosks designed for the average person to operate successfully without prior instruction.
- **Efficiency**—Once the user has learned to use a new product, does the product help the user perform the work well?
- **Memorability**—If the product is used infrequently, is it easy to remember how to use it or does the user have to learn its use all over again?
- **Error rate**—How error prone is the system? The system should have a low error rate, and catastrophic error must not occur. If an error occurs, can quick recovery happen with a device such as an "undo" button?
- **Satisfaction rating**—Do users like the system once they are acquainted with it? Users should be satisfied when using it.

Usability enhances the effectiveness of efficiency with which work and other activities are carried out. Usability increases convenience, reduces errors, and increases productivity.

The process for designing usable and viable systems or devices draws on the knowledge, abilities, and preferences of the user (customer) and incorporates generalizable facts about how people interact with their environment. Therefore, it is not reasonable to expect that, if a device or system works in one setting, it will also work in another setting. When humans interact with a machine, that interaction takes place within a specific context. This context includes social, organizational, political, physical, and cultural milieus. The HFE must consider each of these aspects during design and development. The work of the HFE must begin early in the design process. **Assessment of the user** and **analysis of the task,** which occur before development of a design, and **prototype testing,** which enables continual re-evaluation during development, are important steps in the HFE process.

Assessment of the User

The assessment phase is the first step in the design and development process and is important for gathering information about the users and their needs. "Know the user" is a common phrase among human factors professionals. HFEs do not use themselves as test subjects because their knowledge base and perceptions of design needs are different from those of the average user. If the user's needs and wants are not known, considerable development efforts may be wasted on features in the mistaken belief that some users may want them.

A study of software engineering cost estimates shows that 63 percent of large software projects significantly overran their estimates (Neilsen, 1993, p. 5). When asked to explain their inaccurate cost estimates, software managers cited 24 different reasons. Interestingly, the four reasons that were rated as being most significant were all related to user assessment: frequent requests for changes by users, overlooked tasks, users' lack of understanding of their own requirements, and insufficient user-analyst communication and understanding. Proper user assessment may prevent such problems and thus substantially reduce cost overruns in software projects.

Identifying users' needs in the context of their working environments, known as "contextual inquiry," is vital. An HFE must visit and observe users in their actual work environment, where the HFE can ask probing questions concerning workflow, information needs and resources, and environmental constraints and detractors. When interviewed outside of the work environment, users may overlook situations to which they have become accustomed, but that, if ignored, could have a great impact on the use or design of a new system.

Other clues about users' needs come from "artifacts" such as bulletin boards, brochures, and standard forms. The goals of contextual inquiry are to uncover the crucial product-shaping issues, as well as to set initial usability requirements (90 percent of users will learn the system in 2 hours) (Gosbee & Gardner-Bonneau, 1998). At times, systems designers are inclined to design "bells and whistles" into a system. These features create a glitzy marketing presentation and are eye-catching but may actually reduce the user's efficiency and ability to do the work. Only the people who will use the system can evaluate the usefulness of applications within a product.

Analysis of the Task

Analyzing the task consists of a detailed analysis of all of the activities involved in the task. Analysis of the task is closely aligned with assessment of the user's needs. At various points in the design process, the design team will perform detailed sequential analyses of those tasks that comprise assembly, installation, operation, and maintenance on an envisioned device such as a new intravenous therapy pump. An analysis of task (Sawyer, 1996) usually includes:

- A list of the major tasks, such as calibration, entering operating parameters, attaching the device to the patient, and cleaning parts, or, in the case of software design, the functions that need to take place with each screen view
- A description of the necessary information for each task, user actions, required decisions, and related accessories
- A description of the device or software response for each action or step; a record of observations and inferences about design factors that potentially impact the user
- A list of the effects of environmental conditions and other devices on user interface and performance
- A list of the impact of the user interface on training requirements

Table 4.1 demonstrates a few steps from an analysis of a marketed infusion pump conducted by the Food and Drug Administration (FDA). The initial steps in using the device proceeded without difficulty. The first difficulty arose when the team realized that the pump was not plugged in but was operating on the battery. This was not initially detected because the battery and AC icons were small and poorly positioned. From a distance, they appeared as small dots and were therefore overlooked by the user. Important status and prompt information appeared only briefly on the screen, and the user often missed it. Depressing the flow rate button for more than a fraction of a second caused the numbers to scroll past the desired value too quickly. Auditory feedback was heard after the initial key press, not after each of the scrolled values. Navigation and operating modes were inconsistent, causing confusion. Completing the task analysis early in the design process eliminated the product's inconsistencies and increased its safety, making it more user friendly.

TABLE 4.1 ▶ **TASK ANALYSIS**

User Action	Device Response	Observed Problem
1. Push "on" button.	If unplugged, battery light (icon) glows. If plugged in, power light glows. "Select Mode" message appears for 3 seconds. Flow rate and volume displays show "0" even if there is a default value.	Battery and power lights are so small and poorly positioned that user probably will not notice power status. User is likely to miss mode indication and leave device in previous (default) mode. Many other pumps show default value from last mode. User may assume no default value with this pump (see step 3).
2. Press pump mode button.	Mode light glows.	Mode lights do not blink, are small, and can easily be missed. Each light is close to a key with no functional relationship. Incorrect association is very possible.
3. Press rate button.	Flow rate displays default value from previous administration.	User experienced with another pump may assume a "0" value by this point and miss default value (see step 1).
4. Enter flow rate values in mL per hour.	As first value (e.g., 100 mL) is entered, device "beeps" and 100 is displayed. User can scroll in increments of 100, and successive values are displayed, but no more "beeps" occur. With constant pressure on key, values may scroll up to 300 mL, for example, in 1 second.	A distracted user, not observing the display, may intentionally or accidentally enter more values without any auditory feedback to indicate entry.

Prototype Testing

Prototype testing involves iterative or repetitive evaluation of equipment and software throughout the design cycle. Low-fidelity prototypes are simple renditions of an actual product. Instead of actually programming a series of computer screens, a low-fidelity prototype may consist of a series of paper screens. A paper-and-pencil mock-up can be a series of drawn screens depicting what the user will see on an automated screen, or it can be a picture of a device with buttons, dials, and switches drawn in place. As development progresses, analyses will mature from a paper-and-pencil mock-up of the new software or device to higher-fidelity device descriptions, detailed drawings, and actual prototype devices. This process is inexpensive, easy to create, and easy to redesign.

Developers create real-world scenarios and ask users to "think aloud" as the users interact with the device or software. Developers collect data on items such as time needed to complete the task, number of errors, difficulty in navigation, and misleading terminology. Subsequently the design is changed based on the analysis of the prototype. This iterative process improves the prototype with each cycle of testing and can be repeated many times until both the designer and the user(s) are satisfied. Product safety is improved as hazards and unexpected usage patterns are revealed.

BENEFITS OF USABILITY DESIGNS

Assessment of needs, analysis of the task, and prototype testing produce several benefits, which include cost reduction because of a more efficient design process, rapid design development because the design team is more focused, and earlier, less costly system changes because of the iterative prototype testing. Clinicians are more likely to accept and use products that have human factors design considerations and evaluative processes, resulting in administrative savings, improved decision making, and decreased errors. A user-focused design process provides the means to exceed customer expectations for ease of use, ease of learning, and user satisfaction (Gosbee & Gardner-Bonneau, 1998).

Stahlhut (1995) provides an example demonstrating how the lack of consideration for usability factors proved costly. In a busy emergency room, physicians had difficulty documenting their patient visits. They had little time and were frequently interrupted; the result was incomplete documentation. One solution to the problem was to hire transcriptionists to translate dictated notes, but this was considered unaffordable. A second solution was to purchase a voice recognition system that had recently come on the market to which the physician could dictate. Because the computer would transcribe the words, no transcriptionists were needed for typing. The system could remind physicians of errors, print out the write-up immediately, and store the data for future analysis. At a cost of $60,000, the automated system appeared to be a cost-effective solution to the problem.

Unfortunately, the majority of the physicians rejected the system almost immediately. Within a couple of months, even the main advocate of the system dismissed it. The $60,000 system was placed in a back closet, unused. Two problems were identified in a postmortem analysis. First, the system was hard to use because it assumed that the physician would dictate the entire patient encounter immediately after finishing with the patient; however, the physicians did not function that way. If the patient were in the emergency room for a long period, only part of the encounter would be dictated at a time. At other times, the physician recorded the encounter at the end of the shift. The new voice recognition system did not accommodate this variation in dictation routines.

The second problem was that dictation on the system took 10 to 15 minutes per patient. This was much longer than the physicians ordinarily took for documentation. Later, it was discovered that the system worked successfully in departments that were either much less busy or had customized the system for each doctor so that it followed individual styles more easily and made documentation faster. Analyzing the users and the tasks and testing prototypes would have identified problems early in the design process and saved the facility $60,000.

PSYCHOLOGY OF HUMAN FACTORS

Human factors psychologists discover and apply information about human behavior, limitations, capabilities, and other characteristics to the design of tools, machines, systems, tasks, jobs, and environments for productive, safe, comfortable, and effective human use (Stramler, 1993). The human capability dimensions of **anthropometry, perception, cognition, action, memory, mental models,** and the **effects of aging** are basic to an understanding of human factors.

Anthropometry

The word "anthropometry" is derived from the Greek words *anthropos,* meaning human, and *metrikos,* meaning measurement. It refers to physical measurements of the human body. What angle must the wrists and fingers assume to perform data entry? In what direction must the head turn to see the terminal screen? How far must one reach to turn a dial? These considerations all apply to physical constraints. Some devices are designed to fit a person of a specific height. An example is a monitor above the bed in an intensive care room with dials that are easily set by a person who is 5 feet 7 inches or taller but are inaccessible to a shorter person without a stool.

When designing a workstation for computer data entry, the body alignment of a seated person must be considered. Physical strain is minimized when a seated person performs data entry functions with the forearms at a 90-degree angle to the upper arm and the eyes looking straight ahead to see the monitor (Sanders & McCormick, 1993) *(Fig. 4.1).* Certain features of equipment must be designed so that they can be adjusted both horizontally and vertically for the range of individuals who use them. Some examples of adjustable devices are automobile seats, office chairs, desks, computer monitors, and keyboards. Equipment must be designed to provide for adjustments to cover the range from the 5th to the 95th percentile of the relevant population characteristic, such as sitting height and arm reach (Sanders & McCormick, 1993). Advising and training are essential so that the user can adjust equipment to accommodate his or her own physical characteristics.

Anthropometry and biomechanics are closely related. Anthropometry considers the relationship between the force required to manipulate

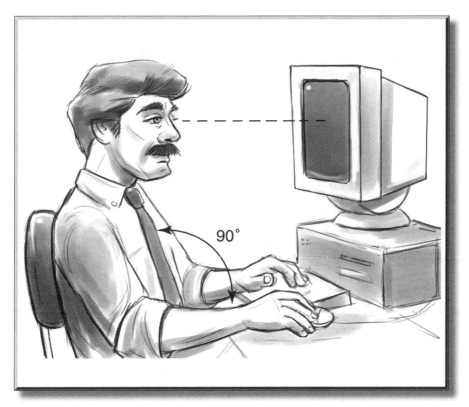

FIGURE 4.1 ▶ 90-degree posture.

an object and the force exerted by the muscles. If a dial is too small for someone with a large hand to grasp, it cannot be adjusted. A keyboard with tiny, close-set keys invites mistakes by people with large fingers. Childproof prescription caps are often impossible for arthritic persons with swollen joints to open.

Perception

The physical comfort and safety of the user are important but not sufficient for good design. The discipline of human factors studies how humans receive and process information. *Figure 4.2* presents a general model of information processing that distinguishes three stages intervening between the presentation of a stimulus and the execution of a response. The stimulus of sensation initiates perception. Following this stage are the intermediate processes of decision making and thought involved in cognition. Information from cognition is used in the final action stage to select, prepare, and control the movements necessary to effect a response (Proctor & Van Zandt, 1994).

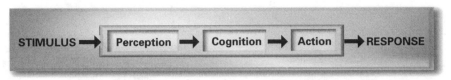

FIGURE 4.2 ▶ Three stages of human information processing.

How humans receive sensory information, especially visual and auditory impulses, is a paramount consideration in designing for optimal human performance. The term "sensation" refers to the initial detection of energy from the physical world. The study of sensation generally deals with the structure and processes of the sensory mechanism (the ear, the eye, and so on) and the stimuli that affect those mechanisms.

The perceptual stage includes processes that operate from the stimulation of the sensory organs through the identification of that stimulation. The most basic function of perception is *detection,* that is, determining whether a sight or sound signal is present. The next levels of perceptual function are *identification* and *recognition.* The acts of identification and recognition involve matching incoming sensations with prior learned associations and experiences. The color red lighting a button on a machine indicates "alarm" or "stop" to most people because this is its common use. Using the color red to indicate that a machine is functioning properly is incongruent with other uses of that color. The color green is most often used for that purpose.

The various levels of perception depend on the strength of the stimulus and the complexity of the task. A small, dim red light does not capture the user's attention as acutely as a large, brightly flashing red light, as demonstrated in the task analysis example presented earlier. Perceptual characteristics are important in the design and arrangement of controls, keypads, displays, information presentation, and alarms.

Cognition

After enough information has been extracted from a display to allow the identification or classification of the stimuli, processes begin to operate with the goal of determining the appropriate action or response (Proctor & Van Zandt, 1994). "Cognition" refers to higher-level mental phenomena such as memory, information processing, use of rules and strategies, hypothesis formation, and problem solving. If a driver enters an intersection at the same time that the light turns yellow, the driver decides whether to accelerate or brake based on the perceptual information received. The driver may decide to store the information in memory while searching the intersection ahead for the presence of a police car. It is apparent that the point of decision making and response selection is critical in the sequence of information processing.

Humans have a limited capacity to attend to multiple sources of information, to retrieve information from memory, and to perform complicated mental calculations. Errors in performance can result from these limitations. Knowing when automation can enhance human performance by using complex sets of rules is an important design function. For example, the complex programming of computerized devices can store seemingly unlimited amounts of information. The machine can far exceed the human ability to store data. Therefore, the designer should develop easy-to-use retrieval systems, taking advantage of symbols and easily understood language for screen and menu design.

Action

Following the perception of stimuli and cognition of the information, a response (if required) needs to be selected, programmed, and executed (Proctor & Van Zandt, 1994). If a decision to respond is selected, then a series of steps is required to call up, and release with appropriate timing and force, the necessary muscle commands to carry out the action. If the driver in the previous example decides to stop at the intersection with the yellow light, the appropriate muscular and mental activities must take place to produce that action. Because selection of the appropriate response and specification of the movement parameters take time, the time needed to initiate a movement will increase with the complexity of movement and response selection.

Memory

Each sensory channel appears to have a temporary storage mechanism that retains the representation of the stimulus for a short time. Auditory signals are retained for about 18 seconds, whereas visual signals are retained for about 1.5 seconds (Proctor & Van Zandt, 1994). Evidence indicates that tactile and olfactory senses have some sensory storage but that the main storage repositories for the senses contain visual and auditory memory. For example, when a message flashes on a television screen, the visual storage mechanism retains it for a short time. The same is true of sound recall. One does not need to try actively to retain the stimulus. The process is relatively automatic.

To retain information for a longer period of time, the recipient must encode and transfer it to working memory. To do this, the person must focus attention on retaining the information, for example, listening for and identifying abnormal lung sounds. "Chunking," or grouping information, also increases the capacity of working memory. Telephone numbers and

Social Security numbers are chunked together in groups of two, three or four digits to aid in memorization. For example, the numbers 975-67-8023 are easier to remember than 975678023. Schneiderman (1980) indicates that if more than seven digits or letters are displayed on a screen, the user tends to forget the first digits or letters before reading the last ones.

Transforming information from working memory to long-term memory takes place by a process called "encoding." This action occurs when meaning is attached to the information and related to information already stored in long-term memory. Those who study for examinations by trying to memorize the textbook and course notes quickly forget new information, perhaps even before taking the test. To be most useful, the information needs to be related to information stored in long-term memory. To recall more information, analyzing, comparing, and relating new information to past knowledge leads to greater success. The more organized the information in long-term memory is, the easier it is to recall.

The use of mnemonics to organize information makes retrieval easier. The Dale Carnegie course teaches students to remember long lists of names by associating the names with a word or sentence and forming bizarre images connecting the names. Many students of neurology have memorized the 12 cranial nerves by remembering the limerick "On Old Olympus' Towering Tops A Finn And German Viewed Some Hops" *(Box 4.1)*.

Impact of Attention on Memory

The concentration of mental effort on sensory or mental stimuli affects the memory of perception (Solso, 1995). This is known as "attention." Human ability to attend to stimuli is limited, and the direction of attention

---

BOX 4.1   USE OF MNEMONICS TO MEMORIZE CRANIAL NERVES

On	Olfactory
Old	Optic
Olympus'	Oculomotor
Towering	Trochlear
Tops	Trigeminal
A	Abducens
Finn	Facial
And	Auditory (vestibulocochlear)
German	Glossopharyngeal
Viewed	Vagus
Some	Spinal
Hops	Hypoglossal

will determine how well we perceive, remember, and act on information. **Selective attention** involves scanning several channels at one time to look for a target, much like triaging accident victims to search for the most life-threatening injury. When given multiple sources of information, people tend to focus on the signals that occur frequently rather than infrequently. Under conditions of high stress, the focus of attention becomes narrowed and only those sensations that are perceived are attended to.

Focused attention is limited to one source, excluding all others, such as reading while other persons are talking. The problem is to maintain attention to one source of information without being distracted by others. When designing a system or device requiring focused attention, competing signals must be differentiated in volume (the more important ones are louder) or tone (a high-pitched tone rather than a low-pitched hum). Color coding is also helpful for focusing on visual displays. Colors catch the eye when the user scans several objects on a display.

Divided attention may occur when one is driving, talking to a passenger, and looking for a street sign all at the same time. If attention is divided in too many directions, performance on at least one task usually declines. Whenever possible, the number of potential sources of information should be limited, for example, not carrying on a conversation while driving in heavy, unfamiliar traffic.

The **sustained attention** used when monitoring a screen for an infrequently occurring signal that occurs at unpredictable times is often referred to as a "vigilance task." Under these conditions, the individual does not take his or her eyes off the screen for fear that a signal will be missed, as with a person observing 12 EKG screens for a 4-hour period. Mackworth (1950) found that the rate of detection of abnormalities decreased over time. This decline is called the "vigilance decrement" (Proctor & Van Zandt, 1994). The maximal decrement in accuracy occurs within the first 30 minutes. Not only does accuracy decrease, but reaction times slow also as the time spent at the task increases (Parasuraman & Davies, 1976).

Mental Model Factors

Based on experience, people develop a mental model or schema to understand how complex systems actually work. Mental models are frameworks that organize generalized conceptual knowledge of objects, situations, events, actions, and sequences of events and actions (Proctor & Van Zandt, 1994). They enable the development of expectations about what should occur. People are predisposed to react to new situations according to established habits and culture.

Internationally, the color red signifies "stop" and the color green signifies "go." There is also universal recognition of the symbols for "male,"

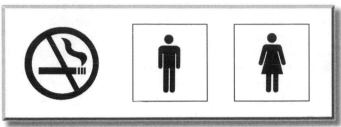

FIGURE 4.3 ▶ Universal symbols.

"female," and "no" *(Fig. 4.3)*. Designs that are consistent with ingrained habits facilitate usability and decrease training time; designs that conflict with learned expectations increase the error rate and reduce user satisfaction. These expectancies aid in the interpretation of specific information and in determining its importance.

Healthcare professionals develop mental models of graphs and digital displays to monitor the vital sign status of a patient. These displays may represent blood pressure, temperature, pulse, respiration, and oxygen blood level. The effective design of monitors and equipment should represent information in a manner consistent with the mental model of the users. To determine the mental model that healthcare workers use as they interact with equipment and devices, human factors professionals conduct studies using interviews, surveys, and questionnaires to identify the model that most effectively represents the users' conception of how a device operates. This allows designers to map user models so that the device and the user's expectations match.

Effect of Aging

The aging process affects human information processing. Although the slowing of perception occurs over a lifetime, it is not especially noticeable until after the age of 65 or so for most people. According to Small (1987), 30 percent of the population over 65 have impaired visual and auditory acuity. Reaction times of older adults are as much as 20 percent longer, and complex reaction time increases to an even greater extent. Strength and mobility may also decrease by age 60 to 70.

Sanders and McCormick (1987, p. 69) suggest the following guidelines in designing a task for the elderly:

1. Strengthen signals displayed to the elderly. Make them louder, brighter, and so on.
2. Design controls and displays to reduce irrelevant details.
3. Maintain a high level of conceptual, spatial, and movement compatibility.

4. Reduce procedures that require divided attention.
5. Provide time between the execution of a response and the signal for the next response. When possible, let the person set the pace of the task.
6. Allow more time and practice to learn material initially.

DESIGN IMPLICATIONS OF HUMAN LIMITATIONS

Obviously, designing out all of the problems associated with human limitations, environments, stress, and aging is impossible. Nevertheless, the cumulative effect of ignoring the human factors of design can lead to disastrous errors. The CDRH (Sawyer, 1996, p. 3) points out that designing the interface with the user in mind usually results in a device that:

- Accommodates a wide range of users working under variable, often stressful conditions
- Is less prone to user error
- Requires less user training

In general, human capabilities and limitations are extremely important considerations in device design.

USER INTERFACE

In the medical domain, a single piece of equipment may have many dials, switches, alarms, and lights. The designer must consider the ability of users to identify controls, interpret signals, and reach and manipulate dials and switches quickly and accurately. The Medical Device Reporting (MDR) system relates that a physician treating a patient with oxygen did not realize that the oxygen flow meter represented discrete rather than continuous settings. Although the knob turned smoothly, oxygen flow was cut off unless the knob was turned to a specific setting. The patient, an infant, became hypoxic before the error was discovered. One solution would have been a rotary control that clicked to indicated discrete settings. Some indication that oxygen was "on" or "off" also should have been provided (Sawyer, 1996, p. 11).

With modern automation, the presentation of information in an easy-to-understand manner is becoming increasingly crucial. Data presented imprecisely, ambiguously, using technical jargon, or in a difficult-to-read format are likely to be misread. Examples of inattention to the human aspects of design include crowded terminal screens, lack of navigation tips, cryptic abbreviations, error messages in technical rather than user language, and time lags between user input and displayed feedback. Serious errors with infusion pumps have been traced to poorly designed alarm signals, cumbersome operating steps, and the presentation of unanticipated warning data on displays normally reserved for other critical information.

The CDRH (Sawyer, 1996, p. 10) offers these suggestions for reducing and preventing software-related and device design–related errors:

- Do not contradict the user's expectation. Rather, exploit the user's prior experience with computerized equipment, and consider conventions related to language and symbols.
- Be consistent and unambiguous in the use and design of headings, abbreviations, symbols, and formats.
- Always keep the user informed about the current status of the device.
- Provide immediate and clear feedback following user entries.
- Design procedures with easy-to-remember steps.
- Use prompts, menus, and so forth to cue the user about important steps; do not "strand" the user.
- Give the user a procedure to use if an error occurs. Provide conspicuous mechanisms for correction and troubleshooting guides.
- Do not overload or confuse the user with information that is unformatted, densely packed, or presented too briefly.
- Consider the use of accepted symbols, icons, colors, and abbreviations to convey information reliably, economically, and quickly.
- Do not overuse software when a simple hardware solution is available, such as a stand-alone pushbutton for a high-priority, time-driven function.
- Consider using dedicated displays or display sectors for highly critical information. In such cases, do not display other data in these locations.

The proper installation of a device and unambiguous indicators of alarm are two areas of the user interface worthy of further discussion.

Installation Considerations

Some of the most common errors reported to the FDA result from the improper installation of medical devices and accessories. Although many errors are not recognized during installation, investigators discover them during the investigation after an accident or incident with the device. Some commonly reported errors include tubing connected to the wrong port, loose connections, accidental disconnection, electrical leads inserted into an improper power source, batteries or bulbs inserted incorrectly, and valves or other hardware installed backward or upside down. According to MDR (Sawyer, 1996), three deaths occurred as a result of the introduction of a feeding solution from an enteral feeding tube into intravenous (IV) tubing used for medication delivery. An adapter intended to introduce medication from an IV tube into the enteral feeding system permitted the reverse operation. Numerous injuries, deaths, and "near misses" with ventilators are also caused by poor tube and connector design.

With the wide array of medical devices and accessories available on the market, designers and manufacturers must identify potential hazards and incorporate appropriate human factors design to prevent faulty installation. Diligence of users in reporting an adverse event increases the ability of manufacturers to identify and correct design flaws.

Alarm Considerations

Auditory warnings and alarms alert the user to problems while the patient uses the device. Although the use of alarms as a warning device may appear to be simple, the programming is actually quite complex. Algorithms are developed to accommodate a multitude of potential actions by the user. Multiple alarms sounding at one time can create confusion and may prevent the user from determining the source of the alarm. Frequent or continuous alarms are often annoying and may be turned off or even disregarded. Environmental noise and numerous visual displays can mask alarms and thus further increase the stress perceived by the healthcare worker. Failure to consider this forced New York City in 1974 to abandon legislation aimed at regulating the decibel output of newly manufactured automobile horns. The quieter horns could not be heard over the noise of traffic (Garfield, 1983). Alarms are not foolproof and may sound a false warning or fail to sound at all. Triggers for alarms may be set at too low or too high a level to give a meaningful warning. Intravenous therapy pump alarms are often silenced manually because they are too sensitive or because the user disregards the alarm as meaningless.

Some of the recommendations for alarm design from the CDRH (Sawyer, 1996, p. 13) include:

- Consider the wide spectrum of operating environments when designing and testing alarms, including other equipment in simultaneous use.
- Consider carefully the effects of oversensitivity, electromagnetic interference, and static electricity on alarm functioning.
- Design alarms so that they meet or exceed the normal hearing and visual limits of the typical user.
- Design alarms to be distinguishable from one another and, to the extent possible, from alarms on other devices used in the same setting.
- Design alarms to activate immediately following the onset of a critical problem. It is important that alarms identify the source of the problem.

- Design alarms so that when they are silenced, they remain silent temporarily. Ideally, they should have visual indicators to indicate status and a mechanism for querying the reason for the alarm.

HUMAN ERROR

According to a June 15, 1997, article in the *New York Times Magazine* (Belkin, 1997), 1995 was a disastrous year for the medical community because of highly publicized errors causing patient death or mutilation. In a Florida hospital, Betsy Lehman, a 39-year-old health columnist for the *Boston Globe,* died not from breast cancer but from a dose of medication four times greater than that prescribed to eradicate her cancer. The total dose of the drug Cytoxan was given *each* day for 4 days rather than spread out over the 4 days. None of the physicians, nurses, or pharmacists noted the error.

When medical mistakes occur, it is tempting to look for someone to blame. Excuses include "the doctor was incompetent" or "the pharmacist was at fault." But more often than not, serious medical errors are not the result of a single mistake, just as the Three Mile Island incident was not the result of a single error. Errors happen when a complicated series of factors come together with fatal—or near-fatal—results (Belkin, 1997).

Errors happen more often than are recognized or admitted. A Harvard Medical Study examined 30,121 patient records from 51 randomly selected New York hospitals. The study noted adverse events in 3.7 percent of the hospitalizations. Of those hospitalizations 27 percent, or 2.6 percent of all hospitalizations, were preventable events. Of the preventable events 10 to 20 percent were system or device related (Brennan et al., 1991). In all phases of human performance, errors seem to be a frequent occurrence.

Various surveys have estimated that human error is the primary cause of 60 to 90 percent of major accidents and incidents in complex systems such as nuclear power, process control, and aviation (Rouse & Rouse, 1983). Card, Moran, and Newell (1983) estimated that operators engaged in word processing make mistakes or choose inefficient commands on 30 percent of their choices. One study of a well-run intensive care unit estimated that doctors and nurses make an average of 1.7 errors per patient per day (Gopher et al., 1989).

Errors are also financially costly. A 1997 study (Lesar et al., 1997) revealed that injuries related to adverse drug reactions (ADR) occurred at a rate of 6.5 per 100 admissions. The postevent costs averaged $2585, and the costs per event for the 28 percent of ADRs determined to have been preventable averaged $4685. Another study revealed that 4 of every 1000 hospital medication orders contained a prescribing error thought to have potential clinical importance.

Human error is inevitable and quantifiable. Healthcare professionals are more likely to blame themselves for errors than they are to blame the equipment. User interface flaws can be subtle, and a physician's or nurse's attention focuses on the patient, not the device. Also, a sense of professional responsibility often prevents healthcare practitioners from blaming the device; as a consequence, practitioners are the recipients of blame for design-induced errors.

Causes of Errors

"People don't make errors because they want to, or because they're bad people," says James Conway, who became chief operating officer of the Dana-Farber Cancer Institute in Boston in 1995 during the institute's restructuring after the death of one patient and the injury of another from a medication error. "Everybody makes errors. Every human being. What we need to focus on is how to best design our systems so that those errors are caught before they reach the patient" (Belkin, 1997, p. 70).

Although problems with user interface do not negate personal responsibility for proper training and careful operation of a device, poor design can greatly increase the likelihood of errors. Such errors can have serious consequences and cannot simply be trained away. "All types of errors are rooted in the essential and adaptive properties of human cognition," writes James Reason, a behavioral psychologist at Britain's Manchester University. "The same adaptive mechanism that allows us to drive safely to work in a state of semi-wakefulness can come back to haunt us when the comfortable assumptions that let us operate on autopilot suddenly turn out not to be true any more" (Reason, 1990, p. 251).

According to Reason, errors occur because of skill-based slips and lapses in which an action does not go according to plan, and rule-based and knowledge-based mistakes occur when the plan itself is inadequate to achieve its objective. Slips occur when the understanding of the situation is correct and the intention to respond to the situation is correct but the wrong action is accidentally triggered. A common example is when a typist presses the wrong key or a slip of the physician's pen turns "norflox," an abbreviation for the antibiotic norfloxin, into "Norflex," the trade name for a muscle relaxant. One hospital discovered its error when a patient's spouse called the pharmacy to report that the patient was feeling weak and experiencing hallucinations.

Lapses represent failure to carry out a recognized action. They are generally referred to as "forgetfulness." A nurse can forget to check the dose of a drug that he or she has received from the pharmacy against the correct dose on the physician order, resulting in a medication error.

Mistakes, according to Reason, result from shortcomings of perception, memory, and cognition. Mistakes are categorized as rule based and knowledge based. Rule-based mistakes occur not in the execution of the plan but in its very design. The plan itself is inadequate to meet its objective. A physician may have a set of logical reasons for determining that a set of symptoms indicates a certain diagnosis. That diagnosis may be wrong based on incomplete evidence, incomplete knowledge, or faulty reasoning. Reason (1990) argues that frequency and reinforcement strongly guide the choice of a rule. Rules frequently employed in the past under certain circumstances, particularly if they have been successful and therefore reinforced, will continue to be chosen. Rule-based decisions tend to be made with a relative degree of certainty, as the operator believes that the triggering conditions are right and that the rule is appropriate and correct. Thus, rule-based errors are described as "strong but wrong."

Knowledge-based errors occur during decision making when incorrect plans of action are created because of a failure to understand the situation. Operators misinterpret communications; their working memory becomes overloaded; they fail to consider all the alternatives; and they succumb to a confirmation bias. The human operator is often overwhelmed by the complexity of evidence and lacks the knowledge or the clear display of information to interpret it correctly.

In everyday life, people tend to practice "context-specific pattern recognition" by trying to determine if a new problem is similar to a problem encountered in the past. At times the familiar response fails to apply, but a prior belief or theory requires strong evidence for it to be overcome. Betsy Lehman and her husband tried to convince caregivers that something was seriously wrong. Rather than stopping and analyzing Lehman's individual situation, caregivers avoided "cognitive strain" and simply reassured the couple that chemotherapy was painful (Saltus, 1995). The staff was so confident that the treatment rules were correct that the error resulting in Lehman's death was not discovered until 3 months later by clerks during a routine review of records. The psychology of "group think" leads to failure to perceive the new pattern; that is, when most members of a group are satisfied that all is well, other members tend to fall into line.

Human Error Countermeasures

Comprehensive training and education are the most common approach to reducing errors. Although training is necessary and can reduce certain types of errors, training alone is not sufficient. Some errors result not from insufficient knowledge but rather from human limitations in certain types of information processing, as discussed in the previous section. Human factors professionals suggest a number of countermeasures that can significantly reduce the frequency and impact of errors.

- User job aids—booklets, posters, labels, or laminated cards can be used for quick reference to reduce the memory load on the healthcare provider performing a task.
- Safety systems.

- Interlock—do the first step before performing the second step. For example, the tubing must be on the appropriate port and secured in position before the machine will start.
- Lock in—keeps the system on until a second action is taken. For instance, the Microsoft word-processing program asks the warning question "Do you really want to quit before you save your work?"
- Lock out—keeps people out of the system until a second action is taken. For example, a password must be entered before access to the system is granted.

The most effective defense against error is to design systems so that error does not occur. In the medical domain, accidental needlesticks became a major concern with the increased incidence of bloodborne pathogens. To prevent needle injuries, the design of needleless IV tubing systems and immunization guns became the answer. Rather than depending on the ability of the nurse to connect the nutrition bag to the nutrition line rather than to the dialysis line, the design of the system should ensure that the connective port on the nutrition bag fits only into the connective port on the nutrition line. Or, rather than depending on the resident to write a prescription with the correct dose of Digoxin, the design of the computer system should not accept a prescription with an erroneous dose.

Industries that have substantially reduced error have created a blame-free environment for reporting errors. Error reporting includes not only the actual errors but also the near misses. Creating a blame-free environment is difficult in a healthcare system trained to understand that anything written down is discoverable evidence in a malpractice suit. The very methods used to reduce error—admitting it, measuring it, discussing it—have the side effect of providing evidence of error that lawyers are eager to use.

Despite all the best efforts, mistakes happen. Careful planning and effective design can reduce the incidence of error and mitigate the consequences, but they cannot completely prevent mistakes. Healthcare professionals must understand that human performance variables cannot be perfected by training alone. Healthcare workers must be taught to modify systems through job aids, appropriate labeling, safety guards, automation, and effective design.

SUMMARY

Recognizing that humans have limitations and capabilities has implications for the design of learnable, efficient, memorable, error-free, and usable medical equipment, processes, and systems. As the use of automation to process and manage information expands and as the healthcare delivery system continues to grow in complexity, an understanding of human factors in the design of hardware, software, systems, and devices is crucial. Certain features of human beings are relevant to the design of the things people use in their work and everyday lives, including people's sensory, perceptual, and cognitive skills, psychomotor abilities, and anthropometric characteristics. These characteristics must be applied to the design of the things people use, such as displays, devices, software, workspace arrangement and layout, and the physical environment. Human errors are inevitable, but with systems and devices designed with human factors in mind, error can be greatly reduced and in some instances eliminated. Knowledge of human factors prepares the healthcare professional to understand why devices and software may be hard to learn and use, and provides the knowledge that allows consumers to be informed in analyzing new products. The selection of products and equipment that have been well designed, with sound HFE, will ensure more effective delivery of care. To meet the challenge of the future in "doing more for less," HFE issues must be given a higher priority in the design, development, and selection of the products used in the delivery of healthcare.

▶ LEARNING EXERCISES

1. Discuss some everyday devices that show a lack of consideration for human factors, such as confusing road signs, poorly labeled products, kitchen equipment without operating instructions, or difficult-to-navigate software programs.
2. What artifacts surround your study or work environment? How do these artifacts help describe the important parts of your work?
3. Write a detailed analysis of a simple task such as tying a shoe or using a can opener. How would a task analysis be made if you were designing a new medical product?
4. Observe the positioning and body mechanics of a worker. What anthropometry issues are apparent?
5. What biomechanics issues must be considered for people of various ages or for those with disabilities in the design of everyday devices? Give examples of both effective designs and designs that could be improved.
6. How does the environment affect attention and memory?
7. What are some common memory aids you use?
8. Give an example of the use of color to assist in the operation of a device.
9. Observe a classmate learning to operate or construct an object, even a toy, given only written instructions. Write down the

difficulties encountered and the mistakes made. How could the design be improved or the instructions written more clearly?

10. Identify how errors and near errors in healthcare could be reported and investigated without fear of reprisal.

References

Belkin, L. (1997, June 15). How can we save the next victim? *New York Times Magazine, 29–33*, 44, 50, 63, 70.

Brennan T. A., Leape, L. L., Laird, N. M., Hebert, L., Localio, A. R., Lawthers, A. G., Newhouse, J. P., Weiler, P. C., & Hiatt, H. H. (1991). Incidence of adverse events and negligence in hospitalized patients. Results of the Harvard Medical Practice Study I. *New England Journal of Medicine, 324,* 370–376.

Card, S., Moran, T., & Newell, A. (1983). *The psychology of human-computer interaction.* Hillsdale, NJ: Erlbaum.

Casey, S. (1993). *Set phasers on stun and other true tales of design, technology, and human error.* Santa Barbara, CA: Aegean.

Garfield, E. (1983). The tyranny of the horn—Automobile, that is. *Current Contents,* no. 28, 5–11.

Gopher, D., Olin, M., Badhih, Y. I., Cohen, G., Donchin, Y., Bieski, M., & Cotev, S. (1989). The nature and causes of human errors in a medical intensive care unit. *Proceedings of the 32nd Annual Human Factors Society.* Santa Monica, CA: Human Factors Society.

Gosbee, J., & Garner-Bonneau, D. (1998). The human factor. *Healthcare Informatics,* 141–144.

Gosbee, J., & Ritchie, E. (1997, July–August). Human-computer interaction and medical software development. *Interactions,* 28–29.

Lesar, T. S., Briceland, I., & Stein, D. S. (1997). Factors related to errors in medication prescribing. *Journal of the American Medical Association, 227*(4), 312–317.

Mackworth, N. H. (1950). *Researchers on the measurement of human performance* (Special Report No. 268). London: Medical Research Council, Her Majesty's Stationary Office.

Neilsen, J. (1993). *Usability engineering.* Chestnut Hill, MA: AP Professional.

Parasuraman, R., & Davies, D. R. (1976). Decision theory analysis of response latencies in vigilance. *Journal of Experimental Psychology: Human Perception and Performance, 2,* 569–582.

Proctor, R. W., & Van Zandt, T. (1994). *Human factors in simple and complex systems.* Needham Heights, MA: Allyn & Bacon.

Reason, J. (1990). *Human error.* Cambridge: Cambridge University Press.

Rouse, W. B., & Rouse, S. H. (1983). Analysis and classification of human error. *IEEE Transactions on Systems, Man, and Cybernetics,* SMC 12, 451–463.

Rubinstein, T., & Mason, A. F. (1979). The accident that shouldn't have happened: An analysis of Three Mile Island. *IEEE Spectrum,* 33–57.

Saladow, J. (1996). Continuum of care and human factors design issues. *Journal of Intravenous Nursing, 19*(35), 20–24.

Saltus, R. (1995, April 7). Medication mixups a growing concern. *Boston Globe,* p. 1.

Salvendy, G. (Ed.). (1987). *Handbook of human factors.* New York: Wiley.

Sanders, M. S., & McCormick, E. J. (1987). Human factors in engineering design (6th ed.). New York: McGraw-Hill.

Sawyer, D. (1996). Do it by design: An introduction to human factors in medical devices. Available: http://www.fda.gov/cdrh/humfac/doit.html

Schneiderman, B. (1980). *Software psychology*. Cambridge, MA: Winthrop.

Small, A. (1987). Design for older people. In G. Salvendy (Ed.), *Handbook of human factors* (pp. 495–504). New York: Wiley.

Solso, R. L. (1995). *Cognitive psychology*. Needham Heights, MA: Simon & Schuster.

Stahlhut, R. (1995, Summer). Medical technology "disasters" and how to avoid them. *AMSA Task Force Quarterly,* 28–29.

Stramler, J. H. (1993). *The dictionary for human factors ergonomics*. Boca Raton, FL: CRC Press.

Wickens, C. (1992). *Engineering psychology and human performance* (2nd ed.). Columbus, OH: HarperCollins.

5

Classifying the Information

LEARNING OBJECTIVES

By the end of this chapter, you will be able to:
▶ Discuss the need for uniform language in healthcare
▶ Define taxonomy
▶ List the benefits of a standardized healthcare language
▶ Describe the need for a taxonomy
▶ List the seven nursing classification schemes recognized by the American Nurses Association
▶ Describe the concept of mapping recognized taxonomies by the Unified Medical Language System and the National Library of Medicine
▶ Describe the need for a minimum data set of information

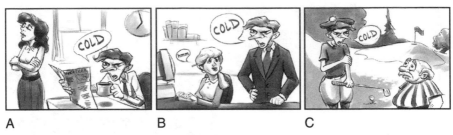

FIGURE 5.1 ▶ Variations of the word "cold."

Early in the morning, a husband and wife are in the kitchen together. He is reading the paper while he drinks coffee, and she is putting away last night's dishes and preparing breakfast. After taking a sip of his coffee, he mutters, "Cold." From this single word, his wife may assume that his coffee is cold, the weather for the day as reported in the newspaper will be cooler than usual, or her behavior toward him has been less than friendly lately.

An hour later, as he walks by his secretary into his office, he again utters the single word "cold." From this his secretary may infer that he is not feeling well today because he has a cold, he is doing cold calling on clients that day, or he wants the file for a client named "Cold."

At 3 o'clock that afternoon, while playing golf with three of his buddies, he tees up on the third green, swings, and sends the ball immediately into the lake. He again mumbles the single word "cold." They deduce that either he is referring to the state of his golf game that day or he forgot his jacket and is feeling the effect of the chilly weather. Any of the assumptions made by his wife, secretary, or golfing companions about the man's use of the word "cold" could be valid because the word has all of the meanings suggested (*Fig. 5.1*).

THE MEANING OF WORDS

The meaning of words is contextually and socially based. The case studies of Douglas and Hull (1992) point to the ways in which a category can be nonexistent until it is socially created. An example of this is the term "child abuse," which did not exist before the twentieth century. Not that child abuse actions did not exist before that time, but the category did not exist and a host of other names identified the behavior. Once the category was declared a legal and moral one, people could recognize the abusive behavior and label it (Hacking, 1986). Once named, child abuse became a reality.

The meaning of a word at one time or in one place, as with the word "cold," is not necessarily its meaning in another time and place. This is just as true of professional language as it is of the language of everyday conversation. "Strength of grasp," a phrase used in nursing and physical therapy, has a different meaning when referring to a premature infant than it does when referring to a 70-year-old stroke victim. A "tall" 2-year-old has a different height than a "tall" basketball player. As phrases filter through the educational background of the listener or receiver of the communication, they are interpreted differently. An occupational therapist may interpret the phrase "strength of grasp" in relation to the ability to hold ordinary eating utensils, whereas a physical therapist or a nurse may interpret it in relation to overall muscle strength.

Two almost opposite issues affect the need and development of **standardized language** for healthcare. The first issue is the development of discipline-differentiated language. This issue refers to the desire to develop languages specific to the distinct needs of each professional discipline. The second approach to language development involves the development or mapping of a healthcare language that is usable and meaningful to the full range of healthcare providers. This approach champions one standardized language for all healthcare professionals.

NEED FOR A DISCIPLINE-DIFFERENTIATED LANGUAGE

Although each healthcare profession shares information with other professions, each discipline has phenomena distinctive to that discipline. Information purposes may differ among professions and may require programs and information management tools tailored to the particular goals of that discipline. In 1990, Chinn wrote concerning nursing language:

> Nursing clearly needs better information, organized in ways that serve the interest of the discipline. The technology to organize and communicate information is already developed, if not yet refined and accessible. Still, the fundamental questions remain for the discipline—What information do we want to draw on? How will we define the terms? How will we obtain the information? How will we organize it? To what end? What are the philosophic and theoretical views that inform and shape the choices? (p. vi)

Roy Simpson (1996) notes that nurses are unable to locate relevant clinical and management information for nursing quickly because of the lack of a universal taxonomy and nomenclature. This lack creates an inability to articulate what nursing actually does or how it affects outcomes and reimbursement. The comments of Chinn and Simpson apply not only to the nursing profession but also to all healthcare professions.

During this time of re-engineering healthcare delivery, many job positions previously held by a distinct profession are merging with those of other professions to create a more generalist professional, a mixture of therapist, manager, and nurse. To demonstrate to those allocating resources and making policy decisions that each practice is distinctive and positively affects patient outcomes, the discrete actions and interventions of each discipline must be named and defined in order to be measurable and to be a reality. A major impediment to the implementation of computer systems to document the work of individual disciplines such as physical and occupational therapy and nursing has been the absence of any unified language pertaining to patient/client care, research, professional education, and administration. Nursing researcher Norma Lang has often been quoted as saying, "If we cannot name it, we cannot control it, finance it, teach it, research it, or put it into public policy" (Timmermans et al., 1998).

Researching a word, such as "cold," offers a challenge. As shown in the example at the beginning of the chapter, this word has many meanings determined by its context and the interpretation of the receiver. Words in healthcare documentation also have many different meanings. Without a precise definition, an analysis of all the times the documentation of the "strength of grasp" phrase appears will show that the phrase has no real meaning. Some professionals may use the term "finger grasp" or "hand strength" instead of "strength of grasp." Those words may describe the same assessment process, but because the words are different, there will be no recognition in a search for the phrase "strength of grasp." Therefore, "strength of grasp" cannot be accurately gathered for research purposes, defined as an assessment tool, or reimbursed as part of an assessment. The establishment of classification systems, however, may eventually lead to naming and describing the work of individual healthcare disciplines.

NEED FOR A SHARED LANGUAGE

Another approach to a standardized language is through the development of a shared language. All healthcare professions interact, share the same overall mission, have access to the same published scientific knowledge, and, to some degree, overlap. In the practice setting, an automated documentation system for nursing does not exist separately from the systems used by social workers, dietitians, or physicians. Nursing uses clinical documentation programs and data sets, such as diets, laboratory tests, and activities common to many clinical disciplines. Informatics assumes an important role in ensuring the structure of data and knowledge in such a way that the larger healthcare community accepts and has access to them. With the use of representative and standardized languages, patients' data can be collected more easily directly from their source discipline and shared among professions as needed for care.

ADVANTAGES OF STANDARDIZED LANGUAGE

Regardless of the basic form, discipline differentiated or shared, standardizing language has many advantages. Standardization facilitates the capture of measures of patients' outcomes from different technologies, such as automated charting, monitors, and automated telephone systems. Technologies are discussed in Chapter 6.

Standardizing healthcare language (Bowles & Naylor, 1996) can:

- Advance knowledge by enabling the study of health problems across populations, settings, and caregivers and by linking diagnoses and deficits with interventions and outcomes
- Promote research findings leading to the development of new strategies for validating diagnoses and deficits and defining new interventions
- Link education and practice, especially when interdisciplinary, more closely through a common language
- Further enhance clinical practice through more effective documentation, decision making, and research-based practice
- Determine resource consumption for administrators more accurately through data to predict costs and the need for resources
- Provide evidence to influence federal government decisions regarding the allocation of health resources and the formulation of health policy by using the available data documenting the effects of care and treatment

A range of social issues, such as the rapid technological development of literature databases, the increased use of clinical information systems in practice settings, and the development of managed-care delivery systems, has created a need for the standardization of healthcare language. This development has profound implications for practice and knowledge development internationally. The development of universal taxonomies and languages that reflect practice throughout the world is a pressing issue.

DEFINITION OF TAXONOMY

Although the term **taxonomy** may be unfamiliar to many practitioners, it means "classification" or "system of classification" (Jette, 1989, p. 967). For centuries, "taxonomy" has denoted a branch of biology that deals with the classification of animals and plants according to their natural relationships. Only in the latter half of the twentieth century has the word been applied to the classification of clinical phenomena. Taxonomies describe the phenomena of clinical practice. **Classification systems** assist in communicating distinctions and precise meanings of words and phrases. As an example, the Nursing Interventions Classification (NIC) organizes 433 interventions into a hierarchical structure of 26 classes under 6 domains *(Fig. 5.2)*. The process of constructing and shaping differences through classification systems is crucial in conceptualization of assessments, interventions, variances, and outcomes.

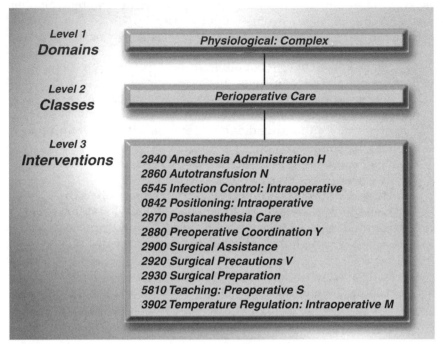

Level 1
Domains   Physiological: Complex

Level 2
Classes   Perioperative Care

Level 3
Interventions
2840 Anesthesia Administration H
2860 Autotransfusion N
6545 Infection Control: Intraoperative
0842 Positioning: Intraoperative
2870 Postanesthesia Care
2880 Preoperative Coordination Y
2900 Surgical Assistance
2920 Surgical Precautions V
2930 Surgical Preparation
5810 Teaching: Preoperative S
3902 Temperature Regulation: Intraoperative M

FIGURE 5.2 ▶ Nursing intervention classification.

ESTABLISHED CLASSIFICATION SYSTEMS

Many taxonomies already exist in healthcare and are used on a daily basis. Most of these systems are medically based and reflect the treatment of disease rather than the holistic or rehabilitative treatments of other disciplines. Common taxonomies are Diagnostically Related Groups (DRGs), International Classification of Disease, Ninth Revision (ICD-9), Physician's Current Procedural Terminology (CPT), *Diagnostic and Statistical Manual of Mental Disorders* (DSM-IV), Systematized Nomenclature of Medicine (SNOMED), and the Health Care Financing Administration's Common Procedure Coding System (HCPCS). The World Health Organization (WHO) created the International Classification of Impairments, Disabilities, and Handicaps (ICIDH) for the broad epidemiological study of the consequences of disease across countries and continents. When studying the etiology, prevalence, and consequences of a disease such as AIDS or the Ebola virus, a unified and standard language serves as a frame of reference for the communication of information. Built on the medical model, the ICIDH does not classify diseases, disorders, or injuries. It covers any disturbance in terms of functional changes associated with health conditions at body, person, and society levels. In the late 1990s, although still referred to as ICIDH-2, the classification levels were renamed to reflect impairments, activities, and participation.

UNIFIED NURSING LANGUAGE

Apart from medicine, nursing has probably done more work to create a unified language for its practice than any other healthcare profession. The burden of learning a specific language for practice and documentation has led some researchers and informaticists to explore the possibility of computerized mapping of language. The primary purpose of computerized **mapping** is to convert everyday language into standardized terminology that can cross-reference structured languages. The system would accept all statements and then classify them. Applying structure to language is particularly useful for research.

Although the need for a standard nursing nomenclature has been expressed repeatedly over the years, no single nomenclature that describes all of nursing practice in all settings is available at this time. In 1991, The American Nurses Association (ANA) created the Steering Committee on Databases to Support Clinical Nursing Practice to investigate and analyze nursing language. As an interim measure toward creating a **unified nursing language (UNL)**, the steering committee has endorsed the strategy of examining and recognizing existing nomenclatures and declaring them eligible to be included in a UNL. The UNL contains but does not replace the recognized nursing nomenclatures and allows each to retain its own structure and identity while providing mapping capability from one nomenclature to the other. *Box 5.1* lists the criteria used to recognize a nursing classification system. By 1998 the committee had recognized six nursing taxonomies: the North American Nursing Diagnosis Association (NANDA) list of nursing diagnoses, the Nursing Interventions Classification (NIC), the Nursing Outcomes Classification (NOC), the Omaha Classification System (OCS), the Home Health Care Classification (HHCC), and the Patient Care Data Set

---

Box 5.1   Criteria for a Nursing Classification System

The classification system must:

- Display clinical usefulness for making diagnostic, intervention, and outcome decisions
- Be stated in clear and unambiguous language, with terms defined precisely
- Demonstrate evidence of testing for reliability
- Be validated as useful for clinical purposes
- Be accompanied by documentation of a systematic methodology for development
- Be accompanied by evidence of a process for periodic review and provision for adding, revising, and deleting terms
- Provide a unique identifier or code for each term

(PCDS). Early in 1999 a seventh language, Perioperative Nursing Data Set (PNDS), was also recognized. Each of the classification efforts makes a distinct contribution to the understanding of nursing language and the eventual ability to codify it and use it in standard ways.

In 1973 NANDA formed and adopted 37 statements reflecting nursing diagnosis statements. The organization now meets biannually to review the list of diagnoses and consider additions. In 1998 the committee approved over 155 diagnoses.

The NIC system was developed to standardize nursing intervention terms. It represents both nursing- and physician-initiated interventions and is designed for use in all areas of nursing with patients of all ages (Bowles & Naylor, 1996). NIC includes the physiological and the psychosocial; illness treatment; illness prevention; health promotion; and direct and indirect interventions for individuals, families, and communities.

The NOC system completes the nursing process elements of assessment (diagnosis), intervention, and outcome. Recognition that the greatest reductions in healthcare costs can be achieved by reducing the amount of care provided produces a dilemma. How can patient care be reduced or eliminated when little is known about the relative effectiveness of different care modalities? The prominence of effectiveness and patient outcomes research made the identification standardization and valid measurement of patient outcomes sensitive to nursing care a major priority for nursing. According to Maas, Johnson, and Moorhead (1996), the NOC structure (1) relates outcomes and indicators by levels of abstraction and (2) groups outcomes and indicators according to rules that define commonalities within the groups. The classification system has five or six increasingly general levels of outcomes.

The development of the OCS began in 1970 through the efforts of the Visiting Nurses' Association of Omaha, Nebraska. It serves as a guide for nursing practice and documentation in home health care and nurse-managed care centers. The OCS classifies all patient problems, interventions, and outcomes. Documentation organized according to the OCS is useful for tracking client trends and progress, billing, reporting to external regulators, making management decisions, and assessing staffing and scheduling needs.

The Health Care Financing Administration financed the development of the HHCC for the purpose of creating a method to assess and classify home health Medicare patients to predict resource requirements and measure outcomes of care (Bowles & Naylor, 1996). The HHCC classifies nursing diagnoses, interventions, and outcomes.

Dr. Judy Ozbolt developed the PCDS; its recognition as a nursing language occurred in 1998. The PCDS catalogs and codes terms in common use in acute-care settings. It names patient problems, therapeutic goals, and patient care orders (Box 5.2).

Box 5.2   Six Nursing Languages Recognized by the ANA

North American Nursing Diagnosis Association (NANDA)

Nursing Diagnosis
111 diagnoses organized under nine human response patterns

Nursing Intervention Classification (NIC)

Intervention
433 direct care interventions organized around six Level 1 domains and 27 Level 2 classes

Classification of Nursing-Sensitive Patient Outcomes (NOC)

Patient Outcomes
282 patient states including Level 1 domains, Level 2 classes, and an outcome label, outcome indicator, and scale and finding

Omaha System (OS)

Client Problems
44 client problems organized as a taxonomy under four domains

Nursing Interventions
Systematic arrangement of nursing actions in four broad categories; objects of nursing activities (63 targets) are used to document plans and interventions.

Problem Rating Scale for Outcomes
Measures progress for each problem on admission and through time
Uses a five-point Likert-type scale for subscales of knowledge, behavior, and status

Home Health Care Classification (HHCC)

Nursing Diagnosis
145 nursing diagnoses coded and classified according to 20 care components

Nursing Interventions
160 nursing interventions and care planning service labels modified by four types of actions; coded and classified by the same 20 care components
Discharge Outcome or Actual Outcome as Compared to Expected Improved, Stabilized, or Deteriorated

Ozbolt's Patient Care Data Set (PCDS)

Patient Problems
363 specific terms derived from commonly used terms in practice, organized around a modified version of HHCC care components
Includes NANDA terms

Patient Care Orders
1357 specific terms derived from commonly used terms in practice, organized around modified version of HHCC care components

Patient Care Goals
311 specific terms derived from commonly used terms in practice
Outcomes defined as the relative level achievement toward the therapeutic goal
Measurements occur over time by use of a six-point scale

Source: Elfrirk, V. (1998, October). What's in a name? The future of nursing (part one). *Healthnet, 12*(1), 2, with permission.

The seventh language recognized by the ANA is the Association of Operating Room Nurses (AORN) Perioperative Nursing Data Set (PNDS). The goal of the development committee was to define, describe, and establish a database articulating perioperative nursing practice that affects patient outcomes. The interventions are based on AORN's Standards of Practice, which are used by operating room nurses in their care planning. Several other languages are under consideration by the committee and will soon be adopted as recognized languages.

As classification systems are endorsed and tested in various practice settings, research findings will continue to provide information leading to a unified nursing language system that describes the practice of nursing. These systems make it possible to include nursing care elements in local, regional, national, and international healthcare data sets (Bowles & Naylor, 1996).

MAPPING LANGUAGE

Since 1989 the National Library of Medicine (NLM) has been developing a **Unified Medical Language System (UMLS)** (Lindberg & Humphreys, 1995). Three types of information are included in the UMLS: a Metathesaurus, which contains information about specific concepts; a Semantic Network, which represents a variety of relationships among the semantic types or categories of concepts in the Metathesaurus; and the UMLS Information Sources Map, which contains more than 66,000 concepts and 100,000 terms from diverse nomenclatures, including MeSH, ICD-9, SNOMED, and the seven nomenclatures recognized by the ANA Data Steering Committee (Averill et al., 1998). The UMLS provides a mechanism through which individual vocabularies can be maintained while making it possible to combine the databases by mapping the terms under which they were coded.

In the future, layered software may be written to support a uniform healthcare language for all professionals. The top or visible layer, written in the language of the user group at whatever location by whatever discipline, is then mapped into the standard taxonomies at another level for storage and retrieval. As of this writing, this type of mapping is not yet available. The companies that create software respond to the demands of the marketplace. The professional community has not yet created enough demand to make the effort to develop this software worthwhile for vendors.

NURSING MINIMUM DATA SET

One step in standardizing language is the creation and acceptance of standard nomenclatures. Another important step toward developing useful data is the creation of a set of minimum criteria that identify the

---

Box 5.3   Elements of the Nursing Minimum Data Set

Nursing care	Service
Nursing diagnosis	Unique facility/service agency
Nursing intervention	number
Nursing outcome	Unique health record number
Intensity of nursing care	of patient
Patient or client demographic	Unique number of principal
information	registered nurse provider
Personal identification	Episode admission or
Date of birth	encounter
Sex	Discharge or termination date
Race and ethnicity	Disposition of patient or client
Residence	Expected payor for most of bill

---

necessary information required for every patient, client, or consumer in every situation. Harriet Werley and Norma Lang identified these for nursing in 1988 *(Box 5.3)*. The purposes of the **Nursing Minimum Data Set (NMDS)** are:

1. Establishing comparability of nursing data across populations, settings, geographic areas, and times
2. Describing the nursing care of patients or clients and their families in a variety of settings, both institutional and noninstitutional
3. Demonstrating or projecting trends regarding nursing care needs and allocating nursing resources to patients or clients according to their health problems or nursing diagnoses
4. Stimulating nursing research through links to the detailed data existing in nursing information systems and other health care information systems (Werley & Zorn, 1988, p. 107)

With the recognition of NANDA, NIC, and NOC, the first three elements in the data set can be categorized through standardized taxonomies. The fourth element, intensity of nursing care, remains a topic of many debates and lacks recognized measuring methods. The Uniform Hospital Discharge Data Set (UHDDS) captures patient/client demographic information, although a standardized, unique patient identifier has yet to be determined (see Chap. 6 for a discussion of the unique patient identifier). Individual institutions establish systems to identify their patients or clients, but that system does not transfer to other institutions and cannot follow the patient from one caregiver to another or from one institution to another. In addition, a unique identifier for the caregiver has not been identified.

If NMDS is adopted across the country, the benefits for nursing are:

1. Access to comparable, minimum nursing care and resources data on local, regional, and national levels
2. Enhanced documentation of nursing care provided
3. Identification of trends related to client problems and nursing care provided
4. Impetus to improve the costing of nursing services
5. Improved data for quality assurance evaluations
6. Impetus for development and refinement of nursing information systems
7. Comparative research on nursing care, including research on nursing diagnoses, nursing interventions, resolution status of client problems, and referral for further nursing services
8. Contributions toward advancing nursing as a research-based discipline (Werley et al., 1988)

In 1860 Florence Nightingale identified the need for comparative data as an aid to producing effective, cost-responsive care:

> These statistics would show subscribers how their money was being spent, what amount of good was really being done with it, or whether the money was doing mischief rather than good. . . . They would enable us to ascertain the mortality in different hospitals, as well as from different diseases and injuries at the same and different ages, the relative frequency of different diseases and injuries among the classes which enter hospitals in different countries, and in different districts of the same country. [The statistics] could enable us to ascertain how much of each year of life is wasted by illness.
>
> —Ulrich, 1992, p. 30.

It is no less important today to use data as a basis for making decisions about effective, cost-responsive care.

Although the nursing profession has been used throughout this chapter to illustrate the use of taxonomies in the healthcare arena, other health and human service disciplines maintain their own languages. In 1979, the American Occupational Therapy Association developed a **Uniform Terminology for Occupational Therapy** designed to present an organized structure for understanding the areas of professional practice. In 1989, a revision of this document outlined two domains: performance areas and performance components. Performance areas included activities of daily living, work and productive activities, and play and leisure activities that are emphasized when determining functional abilities. Performance components (sensorimotor, cognitive, psychosocial, and psychological aspects) are elements of performance that are assessed and, when necessary, areas in which occupational therapists intervene to improve performance.

A 1997 study by Biesemeier and Chima of documentation systems used by the members of the American Dietetic Association determined that the data used most commonly in nutrition decision making were the medical diagnosis, the diet order, anthropometric data, and laboratory values. The outcome measures included laboratory values, tolerance of the nutrition regimen, weight changes, and intake changes. Only 15 percent of the respondents in the study used computerized documentation. The study concluded that dietitians evaluate, standardize, and streamline their documentation to prepare for computerized systems.

SUMMARY

In the present climate of healthcare reform, it is imperative that care-related data be gathered to provide a rational basis on which to make decisions for providing quality, effective, low-cost care. Obviously, automation is needed to retrieve the large volume of data required for this process. Without automation the gathering of data is too labor intensive. Professionals must ensure that the language of care is standardized to the point where it can be reported consistently and computerized for rapid data retrieval. Medicine and nursing have done the most work in articulating their practice through various recognized languages. Other disciplines have made minimal progress toward the development of language to differentiate their practice. Most disciplines follow the path of the American Dietetic Association and use the language of medicine. Communication is best enhanced across disciplines when the same or similar diagnostic classifications or taxonomies are used. Disciplines must either collaborate to develop a single unified language, or a comprehensive mapping system must be created to provide a repository of information that is accessible, consistent, and reliable for planning the healthcare delivery system of the future.

▶ LEARNING EXERCISES

1. Identify language systems or classifications used by professions other than medicine and nursing. If none are identified for a profession, discuss why this is so and the ramifications of the situation.
2. Compare a diagnosis or intervention in more than one standardized language.
3. Contact the NLM to determine how many taxonomies are currently mapped into the UMLS.
4. What research and developments are needed to move further toward a unified healthcare language?
5. How does a UNL differ from a UMLS?
6. What are the benefits of a unified language to a profession?

7. Discuss the implications of a minimum data set for clinical practice, administration, research, and education.
8. Why is the need for a unified language for healthcare more urgent today than it was previously?
9. What are the advantages of a unified healthcare language?
10. What are the advantages and disadvantages of a language unique to one profession?

References

Averill, C. B., Marek, K. D., Zielstorff, R., Kneedler, J., Delaney, C., & Milholland, D. K. (1998). ANA Standards for Nursing Data Sets in Information Systems. *Computers in Nursing, 16*(3), 157–161.

Biesemeier, C., & Chima, C. S. (1997). Computerized patient record: Are we prepared for our future practice? *Journal of the American Dietetic Association, 97*(10), 1099–1104.

Bowles, K. H., & Naylor, M. D. (1996). Nursing intervention classification systems. *IMAGE: Journal of Nursing Scholarship, 28*(4), 303–307.

Chinn, P. (1990). Forming and informing. *Advances in Nursing Science, 13*(2), vi.

Douglas, M., & Hull, D. L. (1992). *How classification works: Nelson Goodman among the social sciences.* Edinburgh: Edinburgh University Press.

Hacking, I. (1986). Making people up. In T. C. Heller, M. Sasna, & D. Wellbery (Eds.), *Reconstructing individualism* (pp. 222–236). Stanford, CA: Stanford University Press.

Jette, A. M. (1989). Diagnosis and classification by physical therapists: A special communication. *Physical Therapy, 69*(11), 967–969.

Lindberg, D., & Humphreys, B. (1995). The UMLS knowledge sources: Tools for building better user interfaces. In N. Lang (Ed.), *An emerging framework: Data system advances for clinical nursing practice* (pp. 151–160). Washington, DC: American Nurses Publishing.

Maas, M. L., Johnson, M., & Moorhead, S. (1996). Classifying nursing-sensitive patient outcomes. *IMAGE: Journal of Nursing Scholarship, 28*(4), 295–301.

Simpson, R. L. (1996). Information is power. *Nursing Administration, 20*(3), 86–89.

Timmermans, S., Bowker, G. C., & Star, S. L. (1998). Architecture of difference: Visibility, control, and comparability in building a nursing interventions classification [posted on the World Wide Web]. Retrieved August 19, 1998, from the World Wide Web: http://alexia.lis.uiuc.edu/~star/nic.paper.html

Ulrich, B. T. (1992). *Leadership and management according to Florence Nightingale.* Norwalk, CT: Appleton & Lange.

Werley, H. H., Devine, E. C., & Zorn, C. R. (1988). The nursing minimum data set. In M. J. Ball, K. J. Hannah, U. G. Jelger, & H. Peterson (Eds.), *Nursing informatics: Where caring and technology meet* (pp. 160–167). New York: Springer-Verlag.

Werley, H. H., & Lang, N. M. (Eds.). (1988). *Identification of the Nursing Minimum Data Set.* New York: Springer.

Werley, H. H., & Zorn, C. R. (1988). The nursing minimum data set: Benefits and implications. In H. H. Werley and N. M. Lang (Eds.), *Identification of the Nursing Minimum Data Set.* New York: Springer.

The Electronic Health Record

LEARNING OBJECTIVES

By the end of this chapter, you will be able to:
▶ Define the electronic health record
▶ Identify factors affecting the need for an electronic health record
▶ Compare the automated record with the paper record
▶ Identify the advantages and disadvantages of the automated record
▶ Analyze the usefulness of a benefit analysis for an automated
  system
▶ Discuss the obstacles to a paperless record

An American woman on a round-the-world tour becomes ill while visiting Australia and goes to an emergency room. Immediately her Australian physician queries the Internet, entering the patient's universal health identification information, and within seconds, through her **electronic health record (EHR)**, he accesses her complete medical history starting at birth. He notes from her history that several family members died from heart attacks. The physician orders a series of laboratory tests, along with a chest x-ray and an electrocardiogram (EKG).

The current EKG is compared with the EKGs on her history and reveals that she may have coronary artery disease. The physician admits her to the coronary care unit of the hospital, where monitoring and recording of her vital signs, intake and output, and EKG is constant. Cardiac catheterization reveals that she has a severe blockage of the left coronary artery, so she is taken to surgery for a left arterial bypass. After surgery she returns to the coronary care unit and is placed on a ventilator for the first 12 hours postoperatively. Medications are administered through an intravenous line monitored by a pump.

Forty-eight hours after surgery, the patient breathes on her own without extra oxygen and is relieved of chest tubes and respiratory treatments. She is started on a clear liquid diet and then is advanced to a low-sodium, low-fat, 1200-calorie diet. Each surgical procedure, and the resulting care and interventions, are recorded electronically on her health record.

On the fourth postoperative day the patient is transferred to the cardiac rehabilitation unit, where she begins an exercise program and receives dietary counseling from a nutritionist. The rehabilitation program and her response to the regimen are again recorded electronically. The case manager determines that she will need follow-up care after she leaves the hospital, and discusses living arrangements and visits by a home care nurse while she is recuperating. Three weeks after surgery, the woman visits her physician at his office. He again queries the Internet, using her universal health identification information, and reviews the diagnostic tests, the interventions prescribed, and her response both in the hospital and after the follow-up visits outside the hospital. After the review he discharges her from his care.

After flying back to the United States, the woman visits her primary physician to acquaint him with the change in her health status. Like the Australian physician, he accesses her record through the Internet, reviews the information, and prescribes a continuing regimen of diet, exercise, and monitoring.

This scenario describes worldwide access to a patient's health information beginning at birth and encompassing all health-related encounters. It also describes the use of an integrated system of applications monitoring and recording the current episode of care. Included in the scenario are applications for the emergency room, laboratory, radiology, critical care, cardiology, surgery, respiratory therapy, pharmacy, dietary, case management, home health, and the physician's office.

This chapter focuses on the automation of information for an individual's encounters with the healthcare delivery system. The informatics concepts of information development, evidence-based decision making, the need for standardized language, and human factors engineering discussed in the preceding chapters are synthesized in the automated record. All of the previous information covered in this text has an effect on the EHR.

FUNCTIONS OF THE HEALTH RECORD

A health record, regardless of its form, has a wide variety of uses. The first use is to document patient care and provide communication among healthcare team members; the second is to provide financial and legal records; and the third is for research and continuous quality improvement. During a patient's illness, the health record provides a single data access point for workers managing the episode of care. All test results and observations should be accessible through it. The record also serves as a repository of clinical thought processes, recording ideas and impressions throughout the period of care. On completion of the episode of care, the record forms the single point at which all clinical data are archived for long-term use. Health records outside of the acute care environment also record preventive care and follow-up of treatment modalities.

CHANGING FUNCTIONS OF THE PATIENT RECORD

In this day of **managed care**, with its emphasis on primary care, with the resulting changes and expansions in the roles of physicians, nurses, and therapists, and with the movement toward regional delivery systems and long-distance healthcare, the critical need for an efficient health record to support clinicians is evident. The managed-care concept has shifted single-focus institutions toward the creation of larger enterprises that can offer a broader spectrum of services and reduce barriers to providing efficient care. New models for managing patients that can ensure a consistent standard of care, as well as good quality and cost outcomes, are necessary to remain competitive. All of these changes elevate the effective management of patient information to a strategic necessity and create new opportunities for the patient care information system to contribute to effective patient management.

The changing **population demographics** are placing more demands on the information capabilities of healthcare providers and systems. The volume and complexity of information per patient have increased. The increased number of per patient encounters (as patients live longer and develop chronic diseases), greater patient severity of illness (both in and out of the hospital), more kinds of clinical data elements arising from new diagnostic technologies, and developments in the delivery system that result in many patients receiving care at multiple sites all contribute to the need for greater collaboration.

Information must be shared among the many professionals who constitute the "healthcare team" making clinical decisions that affect care and therapy. These professionals include physicians, nurses, therapists, dentists, pharmacists, technicians, social workers, and others. Administrators and managers also require information to manage the quality of care provided and to allocate resources according to the institution's patient case mix.

Clinicians need access to knowledge resources for decision making at the point of care. Some, but not all, automated record systems provide methods for organizations to incorporate access to local knowledge resources. Knowledge resources such as literature databases and drug formularies help to transform the data gathered from the patient into information on which to make informed decisions.

Quality assurance activities constitute another form of information need. Accrediting organizations, third-party payers, Medicare, professional societies, and risk managers require quality assurance information. Consumers also are more conscious of the quality of their healthcare and are looking for better tools for assessing the performance of healthcare providers as well as for managing their own healthcare decisions.

Information has become increasingly important to **adjudicate claims** for reimbursement made to third-party payers. As expenditures related to healthcare have risen and as third-party payers have sought to contain costs, payers have also increased their demands for data. Patient data now are used for coverage decisions as well as for payment.

In addition, **data to support research** are needed. Part of the work of the National Library of Medicine (NLM) applies the results of academic research to healthcare. The NLM's extensive work with the Unified Medical Language System (UMLS) is instrumental in helping to gather data for research. The NLM and the Agency for Health Care Policy Research (AHCPR) are sponsoring a large-scale vocabulary test to assess the "extent to which a combination of existing health-related classifications and vocabularies cover vocabulary needed in information systems supporting health care, public health, and health services research" (Humphreys et al., 1996). Because of the AHCPR's role in developing scientifically based clinical guidelines, this organization has long recognized the importance of standard data definitions and of capturing clinical data in structured form. The AHCPR has also played an active role in facilitating standards development. Widespread use of automated systems would not only facilitate the collection of aggregate data in support of guidelines development, but would also make effective dissemination and use of clinical guidelines in clinical practice. The clinician would compile the data into diagnosis or functional limitation statements, interventions, and outcomes derived from clinical care records and would interpret, manipulate, combine, aggregate, analyze, and summarize. The end result would be (new) information and knowledge about care delivery, to be presented to middle and top management to support decision making.

The increasing volume of data collected and the continued growth of medical knowledge have created a dramatic need for information technology appropriate for the task of sorting through all available information, assessing the strength of the evidence, and bringing it to practitioners whenever they need it, particularly at the time they are making care decisions. Often, a gap occurs between the information physicians need and the information available to them at the time of providing patient care. According to Covell and colleagues (1985), an estimated 70 percent of physician information needs are unmet during the patient visit. This gap in information availability at the point of care is not specific to physicians. Information to assist with decision making is necessary for the evidence-based practice of all healthcare professionals *(Fig. 6.1)*.

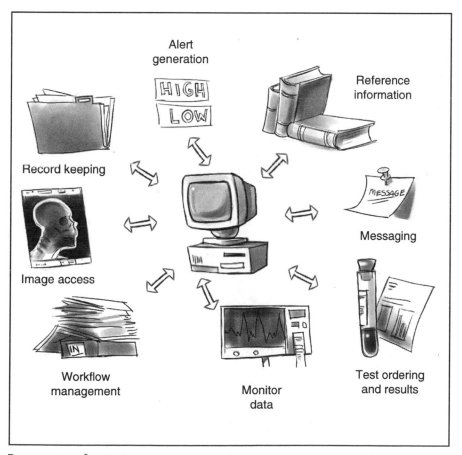

FIGURE 6.1 ▶ Variety of functions of the EHR.

ADVANTAGES OF THE PAPER RECORD

The ways in which paper can be handled, marked, and stored are often taken for granted, but they have some remarkably rich implications. As a physical system, the paper record has many positive attributes.

- Paper and pen constitute a very familiar form of communication and record keeping. The staff requires no training. Because of familiarity with the paper chart system, new employees rarely require a formal orientation to the chart system.
- A paper chart is fast for current practice activities. Healthcare delivery systems for outpatient services contain processes for the use of a paper chart. The typical process begins when a patient arrives at the physician's office and the receptionist pulls the chart from the files. The medical assistant then records the patient's weight and vital signs, makes a note on the progress sheet concerning the purpose of the visit, and places the chart outside the door of the examining room so that the physician can review it before encountering the patient. After the visit, the physician either enters or dictates notes for typing before inclusion in the chart. The patient, the filing clerk, and the third-party payer each receive a copy of the multicopy billing invoice. The paper is returned to the file. If a paper chart were not available, not only the form of communication but also the entire process would have to change.
- The paper chart is portable and unbreakable and can be used easily in almost any location. No special tools or electrical sources are needed.
- The paper chart accepts many types of data, including narrative charting, customized forms, graphs, hand-drawn pictures, EKG strips, and laboratory forms.
- The financial department understands the cost of the paper chart.
- The legal handling of the paper chart is understood and is familiar to the legal system.

DISADVANTAGES OF THE PAPER RECORD

Certain drawbacks are associated with the physical characteristics of any paper system, some of which become apparent only when record systems become quite large.

- The paper record can be lost, incomplete, or illegible. Although it is portable, dropping and scattering results in lost or misfiled parts. Paper is fragile and susceptible to damage, and unless it is well cared for, it will degrade over time.

- The paper record can be used for only one task at a time. Except for a fax, no remote access is available. If two people want to look at the record at the same time, one has to wait for the other to finish with it. Thus a patient's notes may be unavailable for a consultation because the chart is with another caregiver.
- The paper record is passive. It gives no assistance for decision making other than the data entered. In the absence of any formal structure to guide record creation, relevant data are often inadvertently omitted. Tang et al. (1994) studied 168 outpatient consultations and found that data searched for but not found occurred in 81 percent of cases. In 95 percent of these cases the medical record was available during the consultation. The types of missing information were laboratory tests and procedures (36 percent), medications and treatments (23 percent), history (31 percent), and other categories (10 percent).
- Storage is a problem with the paper record, particularly with the recording of large volumes of data. Retrieving the records from storage is also a problem. If a patient arrives in the emergency room in critical condition and the record of previous care is requested, precious time is lost while one person telephones for the record, another person finds it in the archives, and a third person retrieves it. At times, no one can find the record because it is awaiting a physician's signature or for some other reason, and retrieval is not possible.
- Using a paper record for research and continuous quality improvement (CQI) is very laborious. All large record systems require an indexing system to allow individual records or specific information to be retrieved. For example, it would not be possible to walk into a paper record office and obtain the notes for every patient admitted with a particular disease over the last 2 years unless a disease-based index had already been created. The only solution in this case would be to read each record individually to see if it contains the diagnosis in question. This is such a time-consuming and labor-intensive process that it is not frequently done.
- Paper records are vulnerable to error. Because the record is passive, no warning appears if the dosage of a medication order is omitted or a digit is dropped in a nine-digit Social Security number.
- Duplication of information in the paper record is common. Patients repeatedly must give demographic, allergy, medical history, and billing information because it is not immediately available to the questioner.
- Information in the paper record is fragmented and scattered. A clinician must look through many types of data to gather the information needed to make decisions. This contributes to delayed decision making.

OPTICALLY SCANNED RECORDS

In an effort to offset some of the disadvantages of the paper record, many organizations have adopted optical imaging technology. **Optical imaging** produces an exact likeness of a patient record stored electronically on optical platters. It has retrieval, display, and print capabilities. A process scanner transforms paper documents into digital waves by creating a bitmap, a series of dots patterned the same way as the original paper. The image of the page then acquires an electronic format and enables physicians, clinicians, and researchers simultaneously to view records, reports, and results. Because the record is an electronic image, it cannot be manipulated and is known as a "write once, read many" (WORM) record.

The benefits of an optically scanned record include the cost savings resulting from decreased time and labor spent retrieving information, faster service, and increased billing service. The optical image can be retrieved at remote locations and can include video and audio recordings *(Fig. 6.2)*. Optical platters require less storage space, information is safer, and the retention period is longer than that of the paper document.

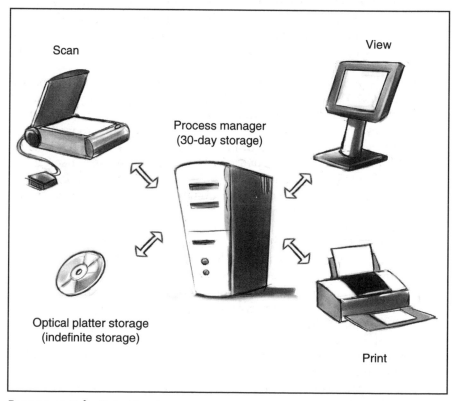

Scan

View

Process manager
(30-day storage)

Optical platter storage
(indefinite storage)

Print

FIGURE 6.2 ▶ Optical imaging system.

The optical imaging system, although an improvement over the paper record, can still be illegible and is passive because it is just an image of the original document. It can be very slow to navigate and allows only minimal reorganization. Because the optically stored information cannot be manipulated, indexed, categorized, or developed into a hierarchy, research and CQI are still laborious.

THE ELECTRONIC HEALTH RECORD

With so many difficulties associated with the paper record, there is a growing drive to replace it with a computer-based record. The terms "electronic health record (EHR)," "computer-based medical record (CBMR)," "computer-based patient record (CPR)," "electronic medical record (EMR)," and "electronic patient record (EPR)" all refer to basically the same concept: a digitized record of a single person's encounters with the healthcare delivery system. In this volume, the term "electronic health record (EHR)" is used because it most completely represents the concept of an automated record for all of an individual's illness and health accounts.

The Computer-based Patient Records Institute defines the computer-based patient record as "electronically stored information about an individual's lifetime health status and health care" (Dick et al., 1997, p. 11). The Institute of Medicine gives a broader definition, stating that a CPR is "an electronic patient record that resides in a system specifically designed to support users by providing accessibility to complete and accurate data, alerts, reminders, clinical decision support systems, links to medical knowledge, and other aids" (Dick et al., 1997, p. 47). Lander and Daniel (1998, p. 6) describe a virtual EHR of the future that is "a collection of individual records that reside in a variety of information systems and locations and on multiple types of media. It contains information from many health-related encounters . . . [that] reflect the current health status and lifetime medical history of an individual. The EHR is virtual in the sense that the information does not physically reside in one place. When viewed on a computer workstation, the EHR appears to be in one place. In reality, the individual records were retrieved from many information systems, such as laboratory, radiology, document imaging, anatomic pathology, anesthesiology, hospital information systems, point-of-care, patient financial services and others. Additionally, some components of the virtual EHR are in enterprise-wide data, voice and image repositories."

The first real EHR applications were installed in 1962, but since then, not one major hospital has fully implemented an EHR (Smith, 1998). According to Smith (1998), the average hospital has 17 separate patient records in its various departments. Each of these information systems approaches the stored information in a different way, and the various systems do not talk to each other. Therefore, no single patient record exists. What is available is fragmented, often redundant, and certainly not complete even if pooled together.

Worldwide access to a continuous health record incorporating clinical applications that all interface, or talk to one another, is not yet a reality in any country (Tang & Hammond, 1997). Most institutions and offices in the United States use a combination of paper and automated records. In some respects, the European community has more records automation than the United States. In the Netherlands, 25 percent of general practitioners' offices are entirely automated, but the systems do not interface with those of other providers of care, so no continuous record is available (van Bemmel et al., 1997). Coiera (1997, p. 66) states, "It is clear that this situation is changing rapidly, as medical informatics develops a more scientific basis. Thus, today it is at least possible to make a comprehensive qualitative assessment of the value of replacing paper with computer, and individual studies that demonstrate specific advantages are increasingly becoming available. Nevertheless, there is still a great need for the development and application of robust formal methods for the evaluation of information technology in health care."

AUTOMATING THE PAPER RECORD

For some, the EHR is simply the computer replacement for existing paper medical record systems. The computer provides mechanisms for capturing information during the clinical encounter, stores it in some secure fashion, and permits retrieval of that information by those with a clinical need. However, merely automating manual records does not constitute an adequate clinical information management system. Cost-benefit studies at the Methodist Hospital in Houston, Texas, revealed that to save clinicians' time in documentation and communication with an automated charting system, facilities "must go beyond merely replacing their paper method of collecting data and find innovative ways to manipulate and use data through automation, a medium whose potential goes beyond the practical capabilities of a paper chart" (Hughes et al., 1997). Automating today's procedures and methods only automates inefficient practices based on yesterday's requirements. One must go beyond computerizing current practices to gain control over the generation of information and devise new techniques for using it insightfully.

This perspective forces a new look at the data that an organization or a profession collects and what can be done with them. This may mean collecting data not previously available, collecting them more frequently, or collecting them from different sources. It may even mean *not* collecting some data. Data that are not meaningful and will not be used need not be accumulated. This perspective may mean improving the accuracy or validity of patient data. It may mean simplifying methods of recording repetitive information or providing capacities for quickly accessing, correlating, and interpreting divergent pieces of information. It may mean changing the presentation of the data, perhaps by altering a form or report or by integrating data previously maintained on separate forms into a common format.

ADVANTAGES OF THE EHR

The EHR has a number of powerful attributes that provide advantages over the paper record. The design of the EHR can address all the disadvantages of the paper record.

- The EHR has enormous capabilities for storing data in a small space. With continual advances in the technologies of optical storage and in magnetic particle systems, this system will provide ever-greater storage capacity for a long time.
- The EHR is accessible from remote sites to many people at the same time. No longer must an individual be in a specific location, and perhaps wait in line, to view a patient record. One of the earliest benefits of an EHR was its improved access to all patient data whenever clinical decisions are made independent of the source of the data.
- Information retrieval can be almost instantaneous. As soon as a laboratory result is entered into the database, all interested parties can view it. With faster retrieval time, practitioners can spend their time in patient care or related activities, not in data retrieval. Thus the EHR helps to save time and staff resources.
- The EHR can provide clinical alerts, expert systems, and reminders. Laboratory systems routinely flag laboratory results that fall outside the normal range, directing clinicians to results that may be particularly worth considering (Fig. 6.3). Computer-generated reminders of the appropriate length of stay for a patient with a particular diagnosis often reduce the median length of stay in the hospital (Shea et al., 1995). Clinicians perform better with reminders on tasks like breast and colorectal cancer screening, cardiovascular risk reduction, and vaccination (Shea et al., 1996). Before each scheduled patient visit at the Regenstrief Clinic in Indiana, the computer reviews the patient's record and reminds the provider about conditions that may need medical attention (McDonald et al., 1992). The clinic has over 600 physician-defined rules in its system. If the patient is a woman over 35 who has not had a breast examination in more than a year, the physician receives a reminder to do the exam and to record the results. Another reminder concerns the use of screening mammography. If the patient is a woman between the

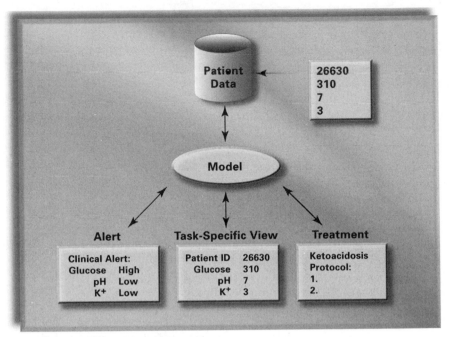

FIGURE 6.3 ▶ Example of a laboratory alert.

ages of 50 and 70 and no mammogram has been recorded for a
year, the system reminds the physician to order the test. The
system also gives research findings supporting the need for a
yearly mammogram for a patient who fits the designated profile.
Box 6.1 is an example of a medication alert and an age-related
reminder. The system also has rules for the use of medication, for
calculating ideal weight and making suggestions about diet, for
calculating the Framingham Cardiovascular Risk Index and
suggesting interventions when the risk is high, for treating
undertreated diseases, for calling attention to new abnormalities,
and for preventive care.
- The EHR can link the clinician to protocols (such as the AHCPR
  protocols discussed in Chap. 3), care plans, critical paths,
  literature databases (discussed in Chap. 2), pharmaceutical
  information, and other databases of healthcare knowledge.
  Accessing can be via anatomical part, body system, specialty,
  date, symptom, problem, or any combination of variables. Access
  to healthcare knowledge and decision support includes such items
  as external references and full-text literature, research outcomes,
  and up-to-date treatment guidelines for illnesses. Linkages
  enable the clinician to access the Centers for Disease Control, the
  Poison Control Center, or the *Physicians' Desk Reference*. Not all

---

Box 6.1   Example of a Reminder System

These suggestions are based on incomplete data; your judgment should take precedence.

Hansen, G. AGE: 60 SEX: F
GAVISCON LIQ prescribed on 09-April-99 is high in sodium and may interfere with blood pressure control.
Consider immunizing with pneumovax because the patient is at high risk (AGE 60) for development of pneumococcal pneumonia.

EHRs contain these linkages, but the technological ability to provide the links exists.

- Automated programs can create customized views to meet the needs of various specialties. Rather than forcing nurses, pharmacists, therapists, and physicians to look at all of the data the same way, customized screens created and attached to an individual's sign-on enable the user to view information specific to his or her specialty. Physicians can then view the information on just their patients for the past 24 hours or access whatever information the physicians at a specific facility deem important. In a similar manner, designating information most important to the needs of nursing and therapy staffs allows them to design the order or manner (graph, narrative, or columns) in which they want to view it. As discussed in Chapter 4, the creation of task-specific data displays assists in decision making by presenting views of only the data that are directly relevant to a decision (Wickens, 1992). Such displays both reduce the effort expanded in collating data and focus attention on important data that might otherwise be ignored.
- The EHR gives information to improve risk management and provides outcomes assessment. It allows investigation of errors of commission and omission, delays in treatment, and adverse events as soon as they are recorded online. Reminders and alerts also reduce the incidence of adverse events. When information on the patient's physical assessment indicating that the patient is at high risk for falls is entered into the system, the clinician is alerted and can initiate risk reduction protocols. Identifying trends early makes it possible to take preventive actions. Data gathered on diet, environment, and lifestyle can be linked to health outcome data, enabling clinicians to address health maintenance and wellness issues with their patients. Collated data can assess the efficacy of particular treatments, determine the costs and benefits, or audit the performance of individual care centers.

- The EHR improves clinicians' productivity by providing information rapidly, without unnecessary duplication, on demand. Providers spend their time in patient care or related activities, not in retrieving data. The decision support and data analysis feature also means that the time spent thinking about patient care problems and solutions is more productive because the information is correct, comprehensive, and quickly available (Milholland & Heller, 1996). However, the results of studies on time savings for nursing staff are conflicting. A study reported by Pabst et al. (1996) revealed that 20 minutes per nurse per shift was saved with the introduction of a computerized documentation system. Conversely, a study in Houston, Texas, found no consistent difference in the amount of time spent in documentation and communication activities after implementation of a computerized documentation system. The study did reveal that nurses charted 40 to 50 percent more data in the electronic chart and that the chart was "more legible, more complete and had no math errors in I&O [input and output] or drip calculations" (Hughes et al., 1997). Chart review required for an accreditation study took less time and was more efficient, saving the hospital approximately $40,000. The researchers concluded that, given the same amount of time, electronic charting was more effective and legible than paper charting.
- The EHR provides more accurate capture of financial charges and billing efficiency. Equipment charges built into the system enable automatic charging for medications that are dispensed, for equipment that is used for documented procedures, and for daily room and service charges. Without automated charge capture, clinicians and clerical personnel must be meticulous in documenting all equipment and supplies used. This is not usually a priority with clinicians, and therefore it is often forgotten in the rush of providing care. Linking the documentation of a procedure with the needed equipment and supplies removes the burden of charge capture from the clinician, making it more accurate. In the EHR, requests for payment from third-party payers are rapidly transmitted, along with checking for format and content errors. Paperwork lessens because fewer claims are rejected due to clerical errors.
- The EHR increases patient satisfaction. Because information from previous visits or clinician assessments is available, the patient does not have to provide the same information repeatedly. Demographic, history, and allergy information is available to every clinician online, and there is no need for repetition. Previous information need only be verified. Accurate and timely billing is also an asset to the patient.

DISADVANTAGES OF THE EHR

In spite of the numerous advantages of an automated record, the EHR has several disadvantages.

- Startup costs for hardware, software, installation, maintenance, increased technical personnel, training, and future upgrades are considerable. When counting the cost of automation, organizations often look only at the formidable startup costs and fail to consider the total longer-term picture.
- The learning curve for a new system of documentation is steep. As discussed earlier, the automated system does not just replace the manual process; instead, it is a totally new way of doing work. This involves changing the organizational culture as well as learning a new way of working. Therefore, several months must be allotted for training and implementation before evaluating the worth of a new system.
- Confidentiality, privacy, and security of the information are serious concerns to be addressed. These concerns also exist with the manual record, but the management of these concerns changes with the use of automation. These issues are discussed in more detail in Chapter 7.
- New hardware that is either nonportable or portable and breakable must be addressed. The use of wireless hardware reduces the disadvantage of nonportability, but dealing with the theft and breakage of such hardware is a challenge for the future.
- The issues surrounding the entry of data remain to be addressed. Who will enter the data? In a manual system, the physician writes an order that is transcribed by a clerk and verified by a nurse or pharmacist before implementation. In an automated system, the physician can enter an order directly into the system. Not all physicians are willing to do this. Nurses, therapists, and dietitians all must address the issue of who enters the data and when. In entering the data, the issue of standardized language discussed in Chapter 2 becomes an issue. No longer is everyone able to enter an open narrative. A standard form of documentation must be accepted and learned by everyone involved with the automation.
- An EHR requires technical understanding to maintain the system. An electronic system may reduce the number of personnel in some areas because work becomes more efficient. However, employing a greater number of technicians to maintain the automation is essential. As the number of technical personnel increases, the amount of space needed for their offices and equipment also increases. Facilities must plan for this as they contemplate automation.

- Downtime, or the amount of time that the automated system is unavailable, is also an issue that must be addressed on implementation of an automated system. With new technology, the amount of planned downtime to back up the system has decreased or even become unnecessary, but in the event of a system failure, a plan must be in place to carry on the business of healthcare.

BEDSIDE OR POINT-OF-CARE SYSTEMS

Determining the placement of data input devices is important when choosing an EHR. Clerical and financial systems are usually office-based, but clinical documentation occurs through either a **bedside system** or a **point-of-care system**. As the name implies, a bedside terminal is a computer terminal installed in each patient's room or next to each bed. The term "point of care" has a broader meaning and includes not only the bedside, but also any other point of care in the healthcare environment. Wireless radiofrequency units allow information to be documented wherever the patient is located. As the cost of technology has decreased, the attractiveness of wireless technology has increased. Wireless network bridges or "access points" combine with antennas that match the unique physical characteristics of each building or floor. As a result, clinicians are free to roam with their mobile units and can expect full availability of both input and output of information. When a laboratory result is needed at the patient's side while the patient is in the nuclear imaging unit, for example, the mobile technology can immediately access that information. Technology has advanced to the point where it can withstand significant external radio interference without serious performance degradation. Security of information was formerly a concern for wireless technology, but security sophistication has grown in the past few years, thus preventing unauthorized access to the network.

Point-of-care systems assume a variety of forms to accommodate the needs of the setting, which can vary from home care to critical care. According to Hughes (1995, p. 146), "most would agree that a portable, real-time communication device with multiple reliable input technologies (i.e., touch, pen, voice), the ability to display all of the patient information, the appropriate graphics and trending capabilities, a quick and easy documentation method, battery power to last at least 16 hours, and batteries that fit easily into the pocket would be ideal for most care settings and clinical users." Some of the forms a point-of-care system can take include a locking docking station that allows a computer slate to be mounted in hallways or patient rooms, hand-held personal digital assistants (PDAs), and mobile devices in a small cart that can move from one location to another.

HUMAN FACTORS AND THE EHR

Addressing human factor issues when considering what type of hardware to purchase and where to place it for an automated system is essential. A contextual inquiry analysis of the current workflow identifies these issues. The paper chart socialization system provides a centralized location where clinicians can sit down, confer with colleagues, access textbook and journal resources within the room, answer pages, and receive and place phone calls from the telephone on the desk. When analyzing the human factors of a documentation system, the workflow and socialization of the centrally located paper chart are important considerations. Changing the culture of an organization by redesigning how work is accomplished is difficult. Bedside systems that are implemented after using a paper chart are not always fully utilized because clinicians want privacy and time to relax while charting; do not want to disturb the patient, particularly at night; and want to reduce the distractions that interfere with charting. If automation moves the site of documentation from a central location to a patient room or to the hallway outside the room, clinicians need the option of sitting while documenting. This may be their only opportunity to sit during a hectic 12-hour shift. After implementation of an automated documentation system, clinicians must be careful not to fall into the habit of double documentation—using paper and pencil to note vital signs or history and physical information before entering this information into the computer. Double documentation eliminates one of the main efficiencies of automated charting. When addressing the human factors issues of work efficiency, the hardware must be conveniently placed to encourage timely entry of information without depriving the clinician of access to colleagues and other sources of information. Telephones must be available to place and receive calls. Clinicians must have telephones in the hallways or cordless phones in strategic locations. Giving clinicians cordless phones solves the problem of telephone access but creates the problem of too much equipment to carry from room to room.

Although a hand-held recording device offers many advantages, it must also be carried from room to room. Some institutions use a hand-held scanner to record medication administration. The clinician scans his or her bar-coded name badge, the patient's bar-coded identification band, and the medication bar code. The time is automatically recorded. Scanning for medication administration can be efficient and can reduce medication errors, but it introduces some ergonomic issues. Hand-held devices necessitate pulling out medications, picking up the scanner, scanning the medication, putting the medication down, scanning the patient identification band, scanning the clinician's badge, putting the scanner down, and then administering the medication. This process can be very awkward. As discussed in Chapter 4, a human factors assessment is essential for understanding users' requirements.

ROADBLOCKS AND CHALLENGES TO EHR IMPLEMENTATION

Technology has continued to move forward at a rapid pace, but many organizational and human issues have slowed the pace of implementation of automated systems for an electronic documentation record. One of the overarching issues is *lack of a common vision* for and *lack of definition* of the EHR. No universal understanding of the concepts embodied in an EHR exists (Tang & Hammond, 1997). Without a clear understanding, users have a difficult time selecting systems to meet not only their immediate needs but also their future needs. If organizations choose short-term, limited-ability applications to meet an immediate need, they cannot move toward a global system of shared information, as described at the beginning of the chapter. Conversely, organizations are unable to purchase global systems because such systems have not yet been developed. Many systems are only automated copies of the paper record. Narrative documentation is far more prevalent than structured text. The concept of a cradle-to-grave electronic record has not been implemented to any significant degree. In the 1998 Healthcare Information and Management Systems Society (HIMSS) Leadership Survey, 23 percent of the respondents said that they had not yet begun to plan for an EHR. Some participants suggested that confusion over definitions generated multiple interpretations. Only 2 percent of organizations reported having a fully operational computerized patient record (Mariette, 1998).

Another hurdle for the EHR of the future to overcome is *usability.* For clinicians to rely on the data in the system, they must be direct users of the system. The systems must be responsive to users' needs and intuitive in design. The Windows environment, with its graphical user interface (GUI), icons, and multitasking, has made computer systems increasingly user friendly, but designers have only begun to consider the user. Progress has been made in understanding the "cognitive processes involved in human-computer interactions in order to design interfaces that are more intuitive and more acceptable" (Tang & Patel, 1994, p. 139). Clinicians need information at the point of care to assist them with decision making. Systems will gain greater acceptance with the provision of tools that help clinicians retrieve and understand data relevant to their decision-making tasks. Systems that notify clinicians of abnormal laboratory results or that link the clinician with literature searches attempt to meet the needs of the users.

The *lack of standardized terminology, system architecture, and indexing* is a monumental roadblock in the progress toward a universal, cradle-to-grave EHR. Healthcare information systems are made up of multiple-component systems manufactured by multiple vendors and owned by multiple entities. To share data, industry-adopted standards must be defined for interfaces between components. As discussed in Chapter 5, standardized languages must be adopted and implemented not only within professional disciplines but also globally in order to share information. Health systems must also have a unique patient identifier to link all the data on an individual patient accurately and reliably. An identifier is often described as an alphanumeric scheme, but biometric technology is investigating the use of fingerprints; voiceprints; and retinal, iris, and facial imaging. The biometric technology records indelible characteristics unique to individual voices, eyes, and hands for identification (Jossi, 1998). The 1996 Health Insurance Portability and Accountability Act of 1996 directed the Secretary of Health and Human Services to identify requirements for the unique health identifier by February 1998. That date passed without any decisions, although more public information forums were held. According to Solomon Appavu, director of Health Information Systems (HIS) financial control at Cook County Hospital in Chicago, the biggest obstacle to implementing this unique identification system is assuring patients and physicians that every computer system used in the healthcare industry is secure and that only individuals authorized to access the system will be able to do so (Paul, 1998). Even if the United States develops a unique patient identifier, this falls far short of a universal identifier. As the global community develops, the need for a universal identifier increases. As noted in the second edition of the Institute of Medicine's report on the state of the EHR, "Until standards exist for uniquely identifying individuals and coding and exchanging health data, the value from capturing and aggregating data will go unrealized and each organization will be its own pioneer" (Tang & Hammond, 1997, p. 14).

Other major barriers to the EHR are concerns for *security, privacy,* and *confidentiality.* These issues are discussed in Chapter 7. As Detmer and Steen reported in 1996, no agreement on what must be done to balance appropriate use of healthcare data and the patient's right to privacy has been reached. State regulatory agencies have defined laws and guidelines protecting the privacy and confidentiality of patients within their state, but federal legislation is necessary to overcome many of the inadequacies and inconsistencies among state statutes. Although laws to protect the security of patient information are necessary, it is in the patient's best interest that the EHR be accessible to clinicians who need the information to provide care. Laws must not be so stringent as to prohibit access to those with a legitimate right to information. Achieving this balance by enacting legislation and policy standards and by enforcing system security functions is possible. In addition to clinicians, researchers, quality assessment professionals, and healthcare managers need access to aggregate data to continuously improve health and the delivery of healthcare. Most of the time, these secondary uses of data can be satisfied without access to individually identifiable information.

The front-end cost remains a significant barrier to implementation of the EHR. As technology has improved, the cost has decreased, but the initial and ongoing monetary investments are substantial. Some federal funds are available to address specific development challenges, but the future of such funding is uncertain. Much of the driving force behind the acceptance of an EHR has been the belief that an electronic record would reduce the cost and improve the quality of care through the existence of better-informed healthcare providers and patients, eliminate duplicate testing, and better coordinate treatment by many healthcare providers. Many of the systems researched, however, are systems created by a single facility and are not commercially available. As with e-mail, cellular phones, and computers, it is difficult to quantify the direct and indirect benefits of previously unavailable technology.

THE FUTURE

Future enhancements to clinical systems will integrate knowledge resources with clinical decision support in ways that directly influence clinicians' ordering behavior. Some of these enhancements will include physician orders that activate clinical intervention plans and interdisciplinary clinical protocols that initiate discipline-specific care plans.

Electronic record systems of the future must offer enhanced communication abilities to meet users' and consumers' needs. The system must be able to transmit data reliably not only to integrated systems within a local enterprise system but also across long distances. Systems must communicate effectively with third-party payers and other health entities while maintaining confidentiality. The report from the Institute of Medicine recommends four conditions for the future EHR (Dick et al., 1997, pp. 47–48):

- Users must be confident that the information they have entered will integrate data reliably from all sources and retrieve the data accurately whenever necessary.
- Clinicians must actively use the record in the clinical process.
- Clinicians must understand that the record is a resource for use beyond direct patient care.
- Users must be proficient in the use of future computer systems.

Until the EHR becomes the norm for all practitioners across all provider settings, the tools needed to manage the quality and costs of healthcare will be lacking, the scientific basis for healthcare will continue to be undermined, and the dramatic transformation of healthcare so urgently required will be impeded.

The EHR will play an increasingly important role in supplying data for computer-based population databases. As diseases such as AIDS and heart disease are studied, population-based data become a rich mine waiting to be tapped. Such data are equally important in studying lifestyle activities affecting the health of communities, such as helmet and seat belt laws, smoking cessation, cholesterol management, and weight loss.

Consumers continue to be more involved in decisions regarding the management of their health and will become more active in using an EHR to search through the health literature, communicate with their healthcare professionals, access data on their healthcare history, track the costs and value of the services they receive, diagnose acute conditions, and manage chronic conditions. Integrated delivery systems may increasingly use an automated patient record that is integrated throughout a variety of delivery settings as a means of attracting new members.

SUMMARY

The patient record touches, in some way, virtually everyone associated with providing, receiving, examining, or reimbursing healthcare services. This widespread use has led to efforts to automate the collection, management, and storage of the data that comprise these records. Adoption of the EHR will serve both the public and private sectors of healthcare. Preliminary research indicates that data automation can lead to lower-cost delivery of services while increasing the quality of healthcare. Despite this evidence, the EHR has been embraced more slowly than anticipated. Major barriers to complete automation remain. Healthcare is a public good, and many of these barriers require national mandates, policy changes, or, in some cases, new legislation. Leadership in government and the private sector must be galvanized to make changes where possible to instigate, motivate, and provide incentives to accelerate the development of solutions to overcome these barriers.

The road to an electronic record has been paved, but it may still take years to reach the point where complete patient records are available electronically to all authorized healthcare professionals anytime and anywhere. Only by capturing primary clinical data from healthcare providers in a way that they can be applied to healthcare decisions for individuals and to policy decisions for populations can the United States achieve its goal of providing high-quality, affordable healthcare for all. An electronic health record is essential to accomplishing that goal.

▶ LEARNING EXERCISES

1. Research a facility with at least some portion of its documentation system automated.
   - What is the present standard for automated records according to the literature?
   - What parts of the record are automated?
   - What professional disciplines document with automation?
   - What disciplines do not use automation? Why not?
   - Who is responsible for entering the documentation?
   - What types of reports are generated by the automated system?
   - Observe and discuss human factors issues with staff. What issues are identified?
   - What does the facility intend to do with automation for the future?
2. Visit a department or room for medical records storage.
   - Are records stored as paper, microfiche, optical disk, or other means?
   - What laws govern the type of records stored and the duration of storage?
   - Discuss the security of the storage system.
3. Discuss the advantages and disadvantages of bedside systems and point-of-care systems.
4. Perform a literature search on how computers are accepted by nurses and physicians.

References

Coiera, E. (1997). *Guide to medical informatics, internet, and telemedicine.* London: Alden Press.

Covell, D. G., Uman, G. C., & Manning, P. R. (1985). Information needs in office practice: Are they being met? *Annals of Internal Medicine, 110,* 596–599.

Detmer, D. E., & Steen, E. B. (1996). Shoring up protection of personal health data. *Issues in Science and Technology, 12,* 73–78.

Dick, R. S., Steen, E. B., & Detmer, D. E. (Eds.). (1997). *The computer-based patient record: An essential technology for health care.* Washington, DC: National Academy Press.

Hughes, S. J. (1995). Point-of-care information systems: State of the art. In M. J. Ball, K. J. Hannah, S. K. Newbold, & J. V. Douglas (Eds.), *Nursing informatics: Where caring and technology meet* (2nd ed., pp. 144–154). New York: Springer-Verlag.

Hughes, S. J., Robinson, J., & Salyer, P. D. (1997). Identifying the what, why, and how of a cpr for professional nursing. *Proceedings of the Healthcare and Management Information Systems Society,* Session 24. Chicago: HIMSS

Humphries, B. L., Hole, W. T., McCray, A. T., & Fitzmaurice, J. M. (1996). Planned NLM/AHCPR large-scale vocabulary test: Using UMLS technology to determine the extent to which controlled vocabularies cover terminology needed for health care and public health. *Journal of the American Medical Informatics Association, 3,* 281–287.

Jossi, F. (1998, January). Fingerprints used to "book" patients. *Healthcare Informatics, 22.*

Lander, M. L., & Daniel, A. (1998, March). The journey to the electronic health record. *Healthcare Informatics, 6.*

Mariette, C. (1998, April). Reality bites. *Healthcare Informatics, 26–28.*

McDonald, C. J., Tierney, W. M., Overhage, J. M., Martin, D. K., & Wilson, G. A. (1992). The Regenstrief medical record system: 20 years of experience in hospital, clinics, and neighborhood health centers. *MD Computing, 9*(1), 29–36.

Milholland, D. K., & Heller, B. R. (1996). The computer-based record. In M. C. Mills, C. A. Romano, & B. R. Heller, (Eds.), *Information management in nursing and health care* (pp. 138–143). Springhouse, PA: Springhouse.

Pabst, M. K., Scherubel, J. C., & Minnick, A. F. (1996). The impact of computerized documentation on nurses' use of time. *Computers in Nursing, 14*(1), 25–29.

Paul, L. (1998, September). Public outcry over patient IDs. *Healthcare Informatics, 17.*

Shea, S., DuMouchel, R. W., & Bahamonde, L. (1996). A meta-analysis of 16 randomized controlled trials to evaluate computer-based clinical reminder systems for preventative care in the ambulatory setting. *Journal of the American Medical Informatics Association, 3*(6), 399–409.

Shea, S., Sidell, R. V., DuMouchel, R. W., Pulver, G., Arsons, R. R., & Clayton, P. D. (1995). Computer-generated information messages directed to physicians: Effect on length of hospital stay. *Journal of the American Medical Informatics Association, 2*(1), 58–64.

Smith, S. (1998). Patient record key to medical searching. *Information Today, Inc., 15*(4), 12–14.

Tang, P. C., Fafchamps, D., & Shortliffe, E. H. (1994). Traditional hospital records as a source of clinical data in the outpatient setting. In J. G. Ozbolt (Ed.), *Proceedings of the eighteenth symposium on computer applications in medical care* (pp. 575–579). Washington, DC.

Tang, P. C., & Hammond, W. E. (1997). A progress report on computer-based patient records in the United States. In R. S. Dick, E. B. Steen, & D. E. Detmer (Eds.), *The computer-based patient record: An essential technology for health care* (pp. 1–20). Washington, DC: National Academy Press.

Tang, P. C., & Patel, V. L. (1994). Major issues in user interface design for health professional workstations: Summary and recommendations. *International Journal of Biomedical Computing, 34,* 139–148.

Van Bemmel, J. H., van Ginneken, A. M., & van der Lei, J. (1997). A progress report on computer-based patient records in Europe. In R. S. Dick, E. B. Steen, & D. E. Detmer (Eds.), *The computer-based patient record: An essential technology for health care* (pp. 21–43). Washington, DC: National Academy Press.

Wickens, C. D. (1992). *Engineering psychology and human performance.* New York: HarperCollins.

7

Securing the Information

LEARNING OBJECTIVES

By the end of this chapter, you will be able to:
▶ Differentiate among confidentiality, privacy, and security
▶ Apply ethical principles to information handling

▶ Discuss how information systems impact privacy, confidentiality, and security
▶ Review several security measures designed to protect information and discuss how they work

A man receives a letter from a prominent pharmaceutical company saying, "Our records indicate that you have tried to stop smoking using a prescription nicotine replacement product." The letter goes on to promote an antismoking product developed by the company. A class action suit filed against a drugstore chain in February 1998 reveals that the pharmacy of the drugstore the man used to fill his prescriptions shared its customers' medication information with a database-marketing firm ("CVS . . . Secret," 1998).

A teenage girl uses her mother's password to access a list of emergency room patients. She then calls seven of the patients and falsely informs them that they have tested positive for the AIDS virus (Russell, 1997). In a similar situation, a convicted child molester working as a hospital technician in a Boston hospital uses the hospital's computerized records to look for potential victims. He is apprehended when the father of a 9-year-old girl uses caller ID to trace the call back to the hospital (Quittner, 1997).

In Maryland, a banker on the state health commission peruses a list of cancer patients in the community. He checks the list against the names of his bank's customers and revokes the loans of the matches. According to a *Time* magazine report (Quittner, 1997), at least one-third of all Fortune 500 companies regularly review health information before making hiring decisions. In addition, *Time* relates that more than 200 subjects in a case study from the *Science and Engineering Ethics* journal reported that they had been discriminated against as a result of genetic testing.

These scenarios are not fiction; they are current events in today's world. "The technology is getting ahead of our ethics," says Dr. Denise Nagel, executive director of the National Coalition for Patient Rights (Quittner, 1997, p. 32). Technology enables the swift and efficient accumulation of information about the daily lives of individuals for targeted marketing, business determinations, and healthcare delivery decisions. Many of the uses of automated information, such as compiling statistics about motorcycle accident injuries to justify helmet laws and providing automated banking, are helpful and convenient. Other uses that invade personal privacy are intrusive and abusive. Most people assume that their doctor-patient relationships are private, but "confidentiality is now becoming a commodity to be traded in exchange for health care," experts warned at the eighth annual Conference on Computers, Freedom, and Privacy in February 1998 ("Database Sharing," 1998, p. 10D). Vast reservoirs of medical information are now accessible through automated technology, but legislation and ethical practice models concerning the use of the information have not evolved at the same pace as technology. Loss of individual privacy is a price often paid for database research for the common good.

There are many more purposes for patient/client records in the modern healthcare delivery system than in times past. In former times, records were pertinent only for individual care. Quality assurance, licensing, biomedical research, third-party insurance reimbursement, credentialing, litigation, regional and national databases, court-ordered release of information, and managed-care comparisons are some of the current uses for medical records. Patient/client information is not used *because* of automation, but automation makes access to the information easier. With the growing need for information, the number of individuals given access to medical information has also grown to include government officials, police, and data clearing houses. The increasing need also increases the necessity to structure how and who accesses the information.

This chapter focuses on the impact of automation in maintaining the confidentiality of the electronic health record. The physical security of an automated system is discussed, and the legal issues concerning computer crime are explored with professional ethics as an overarching theme for each discussion.

PRIVACY AND CONFIDENTIALITY

Privacy is the right of individuals to be left alone and to be protected against physical or psychological invasion or the misuse of their property. It includes "freedom from intrusion or observation into one's private affairs; the right to maintain control over certain personal information; and the freedom to act without outside interference" (Peck, 1984, p. 894). Recognizing a patient's **personal right to privacy** is a form of respect, and mutual respect promotes communication and enhances treatment. Concerns about the privacy of information are not limited to healthcare data. The 1977 report *Personal Privacy in an Information Society* cited consumer credit, depository, insurance, employment, and education data as all needing protection (Privacy Protection Study Commission, 1977). All individuals have the right to peace of mind regarding exposure of self or personal information.

Healthcare professionals have adopted ethical codes that address their responsibility to protect clients' privacy. The American Medical Association (AMA), the American Nurses Association (ANA), the American College of Occupational and Environmental Medicine, and other professional organizations affirm the right of patients to privacy through their professional codes of conduct statements. The nursing codes of ethics specifically address three major areas of privacy: (1) the client's right to privacy, (2) protection of information, and (3) access to records.

Unfortunately, many people with access to medical information are not professionals. They are data entry, filing, third-party payer, and billing clerks; unit secretaries; unlicensed assistive personnel; and others who do not have formally adopted codes of ethics to guide them in making decisions about patient information. All people involved with patient-specific healthcare information must be bound by an ethical code and must have regular training in **ethics** and privacy issues (Milholland, 1994).

Confidentiality is the right of individuals to protect their information or records and refers to the situation of establishing a relationship and sharing private information (Romano, 1987). According to the AMA,

> the information disclosed to a physician during the course of the relationship between physician and patient is confidential to the greatest extent possible. The patient should feel free to make a full disclosure of information to the physician in order that the physician may most effectively provide needed services. The patient should be able to make this disclosure with the knowledge that the physician will respect the confidential nature of the communication.
>
> —AMA Council on Ethical and Judicial Affairs, 1989, p. 21.

The obligation to keep someone's personal and private information secret from the knowledge of others is the cornerstone of the trusting relationship between healthcare provider and patient.

This obligation to protect confidentiality is tempered in instances in which innocent people might be in direct jeopardy if patient confidentiality is maintained. One example of a situation that requires reporting without consent is child abuse. An overriding duty to society occurs when the benefits of disclosure outweigh the harm. This argument becomes more powerful when an HIV-positive person is acting irresponsibly and engaging in risky behavior without warning his or her partner. All persons who have a compelling interest, such as sexual partners, needle sharers, healthcare providers, and mortuary attendants, should be provided with information regarding the individual's HIV status. Healthcare providers must consider the well-being, safety, and rights of both the client and society when determining the dissemination of confidential information. Certainly, relevant data must be shared with other members of the healthcare team if the client is to receive quality, effective care. But relevant information must be disclosed only to those persons directly connected with the client's care (Milholland, 1994).

PRIVACY AND CONFIDENTIALITY LAW

The right to confidentiality under the U.S. Constitution applies only to the actions of the government and its agencies. This right does not extend to access of health records in the private sector by persons, businesses, or other nongovernment entities. However, the U.S. Supreme Court has upheld the concept of privacy as seen in the cases of abortion (*Roe v. Wade,* 1973), contraceptive use by married couples (*Griswold v. State of Connecticut,* 1965), removal of life-sustaining technologies (*In re Quinlan,* 1976), and the sterilization of incompetent persons (*In re Grady*, 1981) (Fry & Havens, 1996).

Growing public awareness of the procedures for collection and storage of electronic information, coupled with increasing sensitivity to the potential damage that can result from public disclosure of some medical information, has prompted public debate and federal and state legislation on the topic. At present, no federal legislation exists to protect the rights of patients whose medical data are stored electronically (Bowen et al., 1997). Current confidentiality laws are fragmented and complex. Federal law targets some health records—those involving drug and alcohol treatment, mental health records, and HIV status—for relatively strict protection, but most confidentiality laws are state laws. Unfortunately, state laws vary considerably, magnifying the need for federal legislation (Turkington, 1997). General health records located in the private sector receive the lowest legal assurances of confidentiality.

In most states, but not all, physicians and other health professionals are liable for patients' physical injury, emotional distress, and economic damages caused by a breach of confidentiality. In addition, breach of confidentiality may subject a health professional to loss of license and disciplinary action from his or her professional association (Turkington, 1997).

WHO OWNS THE DATA?

Great debate has ensued on the issue of who owns the data. Patients desire ownership because it is their information. Institutions argue that they own the data because they provided the site of care and collected the information. Physicians claim ownership of the information because they prescribed the care. Insurance carriers want to own the data because they are paying for the care. Researchers want to own the information to advance the common good. Healthcare information is a valuable and sensitive commodity desired by all participants in the healthcare delivery system.

Patient Control of Information

It is generally accepted that a provider owns the physical patient records created by the provider in delivering care to the patient, subject to the patient's limited interest in the information contained in the record (American Medical Record Association, 1985). This rule concerning ownership of the patient record is established by statute in some states and by regulation in others (Waller, 1997). Provider ownership of patient records does not imply that the provider has a right to use, disclose, or withhold data in the record at will. Patients generally have a qualified interest in the information contained in their medical records. However, the precise limits of this interest vary from state to state (Waller, 1997). The Federal Privacy Act and similar acts in many states provide assurance that patient records held by the federal government and by the governments of states that have enacted privacy legislation will not be disclosed to third parties without the patient's consent except under defined circumstances. However, the "crazy quilt of statutory, regulatory, and common-law rules [that] is often inadequately protected" governs the privacy of patient records in other states and in the private sector (Waller, 1997). General releases that authorize the recipient to disclose further health information for any legal reason are the norm in insurance and third-party payers' contracts. These blanket releases license redisclosure and secondary use of information and result in loss of privacy and confidentiality for much health information.

Under present law and practice, a **release of information** consent is not required for certain conditions. Such consent is not required for reporting communicable disease and a positive HIV status to the public health department, immunizations to a state database, tumors to the tumor registry, and trauma to the trauma registry. Medicare, a federal program, and Medicaid, a joint federal-state program, require the reporting of patient-specific information, but without a signed release of information.

A release of information consent also is not required when medical information is stripped of patient identifiers and used for administrative purposes of financial audits, comparison of cost data, utilization review, or quality assurance audits because they come under other authorization processes, such as the licensing of the hospital or the state laws that deal with quality assurance activities or the accreditation process. Dr. David Korn of Stanford Medical School observed, "If a faculty member wanted to do a piece of health services research involving patient charts or whatever, that person would have to go through an Institutional Review Board (IRB) in order to get permission to do it. But if the management decided to review the charts, they would not" (Hearing, 1997).

Often organizations release and receive medical data with all explicit identifiers, such as name, address, and phone number, removed in the belief that this practice maintains patient confidentiality because the resulting data look anonymous. However, a study conducted by Sweeney (1997) ascertained that the remaining data can often be used to reidentify individuals by linking or matching the data to other databases or by looking at unique characteristics found in the fields and records of the database itself.

Use of Information for the Social Good

As the availability of both health utilization and outcome information becomes increasingly important to healthcare researchers and policy makers, the ability to link person-specific health data becomes a critical objective. With the analysis of large clinical data sets, research can define outcome assessments, treatment protocols, and critical pathways. The Centers for Disease Control and Prevention (CDC) and the U.S. Food and Drug Administration (FDA) can each benefit from the implementation of accessible clinical databases in two ways. First, electronic databases would probably improve patient data for epidemiological research. Second, electronic reporting of events in which these agencies are interested could improve their public health and regulatory activities. Examples of crucial data include occurrences of tracked diseases and information about adverse events related to drugs and healthcare devices. Analysis of this type of data collection for the **social good** gains strength only if individual patients can be tracked for long periods of time. According to the legal scholar Lawrence Gostin (1995, pp. 514–515), "a complex modern society cannot elevate each person's interest in privacy above other important societal interests" such as "improved access to health care, more equitable distribution of services to vulnerable populations, and higher quality, better research."

At present, patients are not regularly informed of this type of epidemiological data use. If all patients could choose whether or not to allow their health information to be entered in a local, state, or federal database, some would refuse. Not everyone wants to be identified by the public health department as an individual with a sexually transmitted disease, for example. With the refusal of some individuals to be part of the database, the data becomes incomplete and the analysis altered. The acquisition and use of personal medical information constitutes a struggle between individual rights and social responsibility that remains unresolved.

Confidentiality Model

In 1989, Gabrieli proposed a three-zone confidentiality model (*Fig. 7.1*). The innermost zone of the model contains extremely sensitive information that may not always be contained in an electronic health record. The outermost zone contains the least sensitive information that may or may not be confidential. The middle zone contains sensitive information usually related to illness and health problems. This zone contains most of

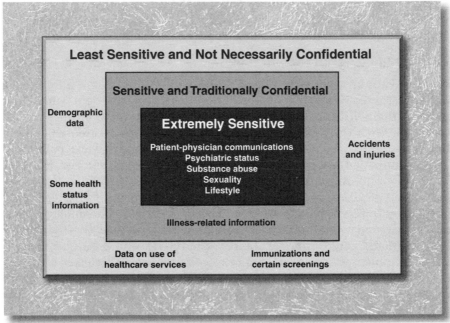

Least Sensitive and Not Necessarily Confidential

Sensitive and Traditionally Confidential

Extremely Sensitive

Patient-physician communications
Psychiatric status
Substance abuse
Sexuality
Lifestyle

Demographic
data

Some health
status
information

Accidents
and injuries

Illness-related information

Data on use of
healthcare services

Immunizations and
certain screenings

FIGURE 7.1 ▶ Three-zone confidentiality model.

the information associated with the electronic health record and traditionally associated with medical confidentiality requirements.

Role of the Ethics Committee

Most healthcare facilities have ethics committees that discuss and make decisions regarding the ethical dilemmas related to patient care. Facilities must focus attention on the important function of this committee and ensure that they represent all professional disciplines when making decisions related to ethics. The committee must make policies and provide structures guiding the use of information and safeguarding patients' rights to privacy and confidentiality. Additional review to ensure that the ethics committee responds to the dilemmas created by the new information process is necessary.

SECURITY

Security is the protection of information from accidental or intentional access by unauthorized people, from unauthorized modification, and from unauthorized accidental or intentional destruction. **System security** refers to measures taken to keep computer-based information systems safe from unauthorized access and other physical harm. **Data secu-**

TABLE 7.1 ▶ **A COMPARISON OF CONFIDENTIALITY AND SECURITY ISSUES IN MANUAL AND AUTOMATED RECORDS**

Issue	Manual Records	Automated Records
Confidentiality	Ethical protection	Ethical protection
System security (accidental destruction by fire, flood, earthquake)	Locked, fireproof file cabinet	Battery power supply or generator Surge protector Offsite backup
Data security (tampering)	No protection	Virus checker, audit trail, access levels
Data security (access)	Whoever picks up a chart can read it, but the person must be physically present to read it	Audit trails, firewalls, encryption, and passwords offer protection, but long-distance unauthorized access can be achieved

rity involves protection of data from accidental or intentional disclosure to unauthorized persons and from unauthorized alteration. Protecting the safety and security of patient data involves identifying the many threats to computer systems and initiating procedures to protect the integrity of the data and system.

Threats occur primarily in two areas, accidental destruction of data and intentional breaks into the system. Accidental destruction of data involves natural disasters such as water damage, fire, chemicals, electrical power outages, disk failures, and exposure to magnetic fields. Breaks into the system involve unauthorized use of equipment or computer time and intentional destruction of equipment or data. Effective security measures are necessary to protect information against the risks of unauthorized disclosure, modification, creation, or deletion *(Table 7.1)*.

System Security

The physical safety of an automated system can be secured through several rather simple safeguards. One of the most important safeguards is an uninterrupted power supply for protection against loss of power. Being connected to a battery-operated backup power source at all times is necessary not only for critical systems that are essential to the operation of the organization, but also for workstations and file servers used for point-of-care applications, monitors, and other medical devices. Supplying power to all systems through a surge protector is mandatory.

Implementing a procedure for data backup is another method of protecting data. Sending a copy of all system files to disk or a tape backup device is the standard backup procedure. Daily or nightly backup provides the best protection and should occur as part of a regularly scheduled routine. Offsite storage of backup data is important for ensuring availability of the data when needed. Backup media stored at the same location as the computer system are subject to the same damage as the primary source of data if a data center is incapacitated.

A factor often overlooked when planning electronic systems is the disaster recovery plan. Natural disasters, such as hurricanes, tornadoes, fires, floods, and earthquakes, do occur and devastate the computer operations of many corporations. Disaster recovery plans are often abandoned as being too costly and time consuming. An outside security expert can assist with a disaster plan and assess the security of the system, recommending any necessary security improvements.

Data Security

Automation presents a paradox for the **data security** of health records. On the one hand, a linked system of computerized health records greatly increases the number of persons who may have instant access to the information. Breaches of security may involve a wholesale invasion of privacy. On the other hand, the technology provides the opportunity for greater control by a patient or provider over access to health information. Digital technology provides greater opportunities for meaningful patient authorization and consent than a system of paper health records. With this privacy-enhancing technology, health information that is transmitted may be encrypted, data can be deidentified by computer programs, data can be segregated, and access to data can be limited to that necessary for the delivery of health services.

Authentication

Access codes, passwords, and key cards are the most common means of **authentication**—restricting automated record access to authorized users. A provider can also use a system that authorizes users biometrically through voiceprints, thumbprints, or other unique individual features; however, the sophisticated technology required for this kind of system may still be prohibitively expensive for many healthcare providers. A key card, much like a credit card, is read into a specialized device that interprets encoded information and provides the user of the card with the appropriate level of access. A **password** or an access code is a collection of alphanumeric characters that the user types into the computer. Passwords can be configured to expire after a certain period of time, usually anywhere from 30 to 60 days. This provides an extra level of security and addresses users whose passwords may become known over time, or who leave an organization but are never deleted from the network security system.

Access

Systems that implement authorization procedures generally attempt to determine whether a given user needs to know the requested information. Great variety exists in the types of information used to develop **access** systems. A common paradigm is to develop a rights matrix with two or more dimensions and assign an appropriate level of access for each matrix element. For example, basing an access matrix on user roles and types of patient information is expedient.

Defining need-to-know status is not easy. Patient data consist of many different items generated in different sections of the electronic record. Each item has a different level of security for different sections of a hospital. Also, different types of professional personnel in a hospital need access to different data items. For instance, the accounting section of a hospital will need to know what laboratory tests were performed for which patients to calculate the fee, but they will not need the test results. Radiology technologists usually need information written on the request form, such as name, age, and purpose of the radiological examination.

In paper records, information is confined to a paper file; therefore, physical control of the paper file is considered sufficient for security. But in the case of electronic records, the data are stored in a computer that potentially can be accessed from any section of the hospital. Technologies to control access may have different layers of access privilege associated with the identification of the user and the authentication of a password.

The presence of an information system makes the physical boundary of a hospital obscure. For instance, university hospitals have research areas and educational areas such as classrooms. These areas are not usually regarded as a hospital, but doctors at university hospitals take care of patients at a certain time, teach students in a classroom at another time, and do laboratory research at still other times. They may receive a call taking them from the ward during the classroom period or in the middle of their research. In such cases, it is natural that the physicians may want to access patient data from the classroom or laboratory. It is easy to install a computer terminal in those areas, but is it safe to allow such access?

After going home, the physician may be called by the hospital regarding the patient's treatment. Again, it is natural for the physician to want to see the patient data at home. A modem connecting the physician at home to the patient's hospital record is technologically easy, but is this efficient access safe?

Technology through the use of a secure server with password and encryption protection ensures that the information is secure from unauthorized access. Responsibility for securing access to the computer screen or any printed information lies with each professional user.

Audits

Paper documentation systems are vulnerable because there is no way to detect unauthorized access. A popular mechanism employed by many computer systems to track access to confidential documents is an **audit trail**. As users attempt to sign on to a computer, the system tracks the sign-on attempts and can even identify which applications and data an individual has accessed. The problem is that audit trails can provide a voluminous amount of information that must be reviewed manually to detect variances from normal system use. Many facilities do not have the human resources or the time to monitor audit trails.

Audit trails provide three forms of protection. First, the existence of an audit trail acts as a powerful deterrent to unauthorized access. Informing users that the system flags each record they access along with their names and refusing access to the system without the system administrator's knowledge inhibit unauthorized use. Users are also informed that unauthorized access is grounds for immediate termination of employment or prosecution.

Second, the computer's ability to detect unauthorized access immediately may permit management (or the patient) to take remedial action to protect the patient from the ill effects of unauthorized access by confiscating unauthorized copies of records before they can be used to harm the patient.

Third, the audit trail is discoverable by a court of law. The audit trail reveals both the unauthorized access and the identity of the person committing the violation. Such evidence can be used in litigation by the patient who seeks compensation for any damages inflicted by privacy violation.

Firewalls

A **firewall** is a combination of hardware and software that forms a barrier between systems or different parts of a single system to protect those systems or parts from unauthorized access. Firewalls screen traffic and allow only approved transactions to pass through them. They also restrict access to other systems or sensitive data such as client information, payroll, or personnel data. Multiple firewalls can increase protection.

Encryption

Encryption is the process that transforms an unenciphered message into an enciphered message according to a key (Sardinas & Muldoon, 1998). Data transmitted over telecommunications lines and data stored within the computer or on auxiliary storage devices like external disks, tapes, or CD-ROMs can be encrypted. The purpose of encryption is to render the data unintelligible to all but the intended recipient. Although encryption in conjunction with security policies could control access to specific components of information, it could double or triple the cost of the system (Mills, 1997).

Confidentiality Statements

Organizations have adopted **confidentiality statements** that all personnel must sign acknowledging that passwords, access codes, and key cards are confidential and used only for patient care. Individuals should not share passwords or leave terminals logged in and unattended. To discourage password and access code sharing, an individual needs to be available 24 hours a day to assist authorized users who forget their access codes and persons with a legitimate need of one-time record access.

Many confidentiality statements are limited to patient data and do not specifically address areas related to computer and network utilization. A systems use policy focused on patient information access and employee records access, as well as computer and network utilization, can be an effective means of communicating specific organizational expectations related to maintaining security and confidentiality.

COMPUTER CRIME

Even the best-secured systems can be penetrated (Hebda et al., 1998). Although more laws are being enacted to define **computer crime,** it is still difficult to detect and prosecute. Although the following terms are not exclusive to healthcare, they are all applicable to the healthcare environment (Hebda et al., 1998; Joos et al., 1992).

Terms Related to Computer Crime

Cracker: A term often confused with "hacker." A cracker enters a computer system illegally and creates mischief.

Hacker: An individual who has average or above-average knowledge of computer technology and who dislikes rules and restrictions. Hackers penetrate systems as a challenge, and many do not regard their acts as criminal.

Logic or Time Bombs: Instructions in a program that performs certain functions on a specific date or at a specific time: for example, printing out information triggered by a specific date, user name, account name, or time.

Sabotage: Destruction of computer equipment or records or disruption of normal system operation. Sabotage can be carried out by both insiders and outsiders and by both authorized and unauthorized system users. Software vendors have been known to sabotage a system when payment has been withheld for a system's failure to meet contractual standards (Waller, 1997).

Trojan Horse: A program that appears to perform one action, but it actually performs another, undesired function. Common examples are replacing a system log-in with another person's password or printing out information every time information on a certain diagnosis is entered.

Virus: A program written deliberately to infect a program and replicate itself to cause damage.

Worm: Like a virus, a program written to replicate itself within another program. When activated, it self-replicates, filling up the computer system so that other applications are compromised.

Providers using computer-based record systems have a legal obligation to take security measures that are reasonable, at least by current standards. One catastrophic incident involving a computer-based patient record system could set the legal status of computer-based records back decades. Therefore, development of improved security technology is of the utmost importance.

Laws and Policies

Computer crime is difficult to prosecute because it is often undetected and unreported. In addition, the passage of laws protecting computerized information has not kept pace with technology. When data are stolen, they are not always seen as valuable and thus the crime is not prosecuted. Most of the federal laws concerning data address only data in federal institutions. The Freedom of Information Act of 1970 allows citizens to access data gathered by federal agencies. The Federal Privacy Act of 1974 stipulates that there can be no secret personnel files; individuals must be allowed to know what is stored in files about them and how it is used. It further ensures that patient information will not be released to third parties without the knowledge and consent of the patient except under defined circumstances. The Computer Fraud and Abuse Act of 1984, amended in 1986, makes it a crime to access a federal computer without authorization and to alter, destroy, or damage information or prevent authorized access.

Two laws that protect all citizens are the Electronic Communication Privacy Act of 1986 and the U.S. Copyright Law. The former protects all citizens from surreptitious interception of wire, oral, or electronic communication. The latter stipulates that it is a federal offense to reproduce computer software without authorization.

The Health Insurance Portability and Accountability Act of 1996 directs the Secretary of Health and Human Services to adopt standards to simplify administrative practices, such as eligibility, enrollment, and remittance in health plans, and to protect the privacy of individually identifiable health information (Health Insurance . . . Act, 1996).

As of this writing, no new legislation has resulted from this directive.

ROLE OF HEALTHCARE PROFESSIONALS

Many beneficial changes can be implemented by persons closest to the technology and the provision of healthcare. What is needed is the encouragement of a climate in which privacy-supportive innovation grows. Informing health professionals about legislation concerning automation issues and becoming active on ethics and other committees to govern the use of and access to patient information are necessary. The challenge is to design a reformed electronic health record system that will protect and even enhance the most important health values while not ignoring other values important to human dignity and the right to privacy.

Fry and Havens (1996, p. 267) underscore the importance of reaching a consensus on a standard of care. "Before we can agree on a standard of care, the various care standards already being maintained by current health care plans need to be discussed and subjected to ethical analysis. . . . [B]efore additional proposals are placed before us, we need more information about the present status of health care in this country and the various health care delivery systems through which care is provided." All health professionals must be active in designing and implementing standards to assess the outcomes and cost effectiveness of healthcare while maintaining the privacy and confidentiality of patient information.

SUMMARY

This is a very important period for health records confidentiality. With the restructuring of health payment systems, the computerization of health records, and the economic priority of cost containment, there is an urgent need to enact national legislation that will regulate access to personal health information. In the rush to develop and assess policy on complex issues, there is a risk that the values of confidentiality and privacy will not play a central role in national policy.

Protecting privacy through confidentiality policies and technology is a critical component of quality healthcare. Legal assurances of confidentiality and privacy demonstrate respect for the autonomy of the patient and encourage participation in the healthcare delivery system and scientific research. "The unprecedented capacity of digital technology to acquire, merge, and disseminate data instantaneously encourages euphoria about the benefits of the technology, cynicism about the relevance of traditional privacy and confidentiality values, and fatalism about the future of privacy and confidentiality. Cynicism and fatalism about the incompatibility of privacy and confidentiality and information technology ought not be an important part of national policy. If information technology overwhelms privacy and confidentiality, it will be because we lack political will, not because of the inevitable consequences of the new technology or of healthcare economics" (Turkington, 1997, p. 126).

All health professionals must be involved both locally and nationally in the processes that affect the confidentiality and security of patient data. Keeping one's password confidential and not discussing patients in the hearing of unauthorized persons are no longer the professional limits of ethical behavior. Active involvement in the decision-making processes of information handling is required. Protecting patients' privacy preserves their right to have information about their health so that they can make choices based on their own values, not on the values of healthcare professionals.

▶ LEARNING EXERCISES

1. What effect do current release-of-information laws and practices have on the concept of the cradle-to-grave electronic health record?
2. Research the release-of-information practices at a local agency or institution. Ask the following questions:
   - Is there one consistent release-of-information policy or does each sector set its own?
   - Which contracts and agreements affect release of patient information?
   - Does the facility allow outside agencies to review the medical records of hospitalized patients?
   - How do the departments of risk management, quality management, and utilization management handle the release of information?
   - What function does the ethics committee have in regard to the release of information?
   - Are other departments releasing patient information?
   - Is there an attorney to contact for legal advice on specific facts and problems?
3. When thinking about individual rights versus social good, if one does not want to share one's personal care data, even with the

assurance that personal identifiers will be stripped from the records, should one be able to access the healthcare knowledge that is developed through the use of the data of others?

4. Compare the security of the paper record to the security of the electronic record.

5. What disaster recovery plans relating to automated information are in place at local facilities that have electronic records?

References

American Medical Association Council on Ethical and Judicial Affairs. (1989). *Current opinions.* Chicago: American Medical Association.

American Medical Record Association. (1985). Position statement, confidentiality of patient health information. In *Accreditation manual for hospitals (1990).* Chicago: Joint Commission on Accreditation of Healthcare Organizations (MR 3.1).

Bowen, J. W., Klimczak, C., Ruiz, M., & Barnes, M. (1997). Design of access control methods for protecting the confidentiality of patient information in networked systems. *Proceedings of the American Medical Informatics Association annual fall symposium,* 46–50.

CVS can't keep a secret; customer sues for breach of confidentiality. (1998, March 29). *Kalamazoo Gazette,* p. E4.

Database sharing eroding medical confidentiality. (1998, February 23). *USA Today,* p. 10D.

Fry, S. T., & Havens, G. A. (1996). Ethical issues in the management of patient data: Maintaining confidentiality in a reformed health care system. In M. C. Mills, C. A. Romano, & B. R. Heller (Eds.), *Information management in nursing and health care* (pp. 257–263). Springhouse, PA: Springhouse.

Gabrieli, E. R. (1989). Electronic ambulatory medical record. *Journal of Clinical Computing, 18*(2), 27–53.

Gostin, L. O. (1995). Health information privacy. *Cornell Law Review, 80,* 514–515.

Health Insurance Portability and Accountability Act of 1996, P. L. No. 104–191, 110 Stat. 1936.

Hearing of the National Committee on Vital and Health Statistics of the 105th Congress Subcommittee on Confidentiality and Privacy (1997, January 13). Online at http://aspe.os.dhhs.gov/ncvhs/privrecs.htm. Visited July 24, 1997.

Hebda, T., Czar, P., & Mascara, C. (1998). *Handbook of informatics for nurses & health care professionals,* Menlo Park, CA: Addison-Wesley.

Joos, I., Whitman, N. I., Smith, M. J., & Nelson, R. (1992). *Computers in small bytes.* New York: National League for Nursing Press.

Milholland, K. (1994). Privacy and confidentiality of patient information. *JONA, 24*(2), 19–24.

Mills, M. E. (1997). Data privacy and confidentiality in the public arena. *Proceedings of the American Medical Informatics Association annual fall symposium,* 42–44.

Peck, R. S. (1984). Extending the constitutional right to privacy in the new technological age. *Hofstra Law Review, 12,* 893–912.

Privacy Protection Study Commission. (1977). *Personal privacy in an information society.* Washington, DC: U.S. Government Printing Office.

Quittner, J. (1997, August 25). Invasion of privacy. *Time*, pp. 30–35.

Romano, C. (1987). Confidentiality and security of computerized systems: The nursing responsibility. *Computers in Nursing, 5*(3), 99–104.

Russell, S. L. (1997). Maintaining data integrity. In N. A. Krieider & B. J. Haselton (Eds.), *The systems challenge* (pp. 177–187). Chicago: American Hospital Association.

Sardinas, J. L., & Muldoon, J. D. (1998). Securing the transmission and storage of medical information. *Computers in Nursing, 16*(3), 162–168.

Sweeney, L. (1997). Guaranteeing anonymity when sharing medical data, the Datafly System. *Proceedings of the American Medical Informatics Association annual fall symposium,* 51–55.

Turkington, R. C. (1997). Medical record confidentiality law, scientific research, and data collection in the information age. *Journal of Law, Medicine & Ethics, 25,* 113–129.

Waller, A. A. (1997). Legal aspects of computer-based patient records and record systems. In D. E. Detmer, E. B. Steen, & R. S. Dick (Eds.), *The computer-based patient record* (pp. 200–223). Washington, DC: National Academy Press.

Changing the Information System

LEARNING OBJECTIVES

By the end of this chapter, you will be able to:
▶ Explain the impact of computer-based information systems on organizations
▶ Explain the importance of organizational culture in system implementation
▶ Define and describe organizational culture

▶ Analyze the importance of culture when implementing information technology
▶ Identify Lewin's three stages of change
▶ Identify Rogers's innovation adopter categories
▶ Apply Lewin's stages of change and Rogers's adopter categories to change situation
▶ Articulate the role of healthcare professionals in managing change

The president of a large home health organization decides to centralize and automate the 270 offices of his operations in 43 states. He envisions taking in client information, scheduling employees, and billing clients as processes similar to those of an airlines reservations system. Routing all calls to one large, centralized office, employees could enter client information into a database. An automated system could match the client's needs to the appropriate caregiver and, using the automated scheduling system, dispatch the caregiver to the client's home. Billing would result from the computer-scheduled visit.

The president's plan sounds feasible, efficient, and cutting edge to the board of directors, which authorizes $25 million for the project. Part of the appeal of the plan is the projected cost saving resulting from the elimination of the small local offices scattered around the country, each with its own office staff, overhead, and equipment.

To prevent rumors of employee layoffs and to conceal the plan from the competition, the designing and planning of the project are secret. Offices for the 50 project team members are located in a building separate from corporate headquarters. Contact between project team members and employees in the field is limited. In addition to the programmers, one expert from billing, one from scheduling, one from human resources, and one from nursing are on the team.

The project director gives updates about the project only to the board of directors, describing the exciting progress of software development and testing. Designing new processes for automated billing of state and federal agencies keeps the excitement running high. Project leaders crisscross the country to sell the new concepts to government agencies. New work processes are designed and job descriptions written to outline a new way of doing the work of the home health industry.

During trial testing the new technology performs admirably. Everything works as designed. The first major difficulties arise as data on current clients and employees sent from local offices to the pilot site prove inaccurate and incomplete. In an effort to avoid the syndrome of "garbage in, garbage out," project team members travel to the local offices to gather the hard-copy data, bring them back to the pilot office, and enter them into the database. This proves to be a time-consuming task met with hostility in offices. In some cases, employees knowing they are losing their jobs have sabotaged the information.

To test the new way of doing work, five local offices turn their operations over to the centralized pilot site. Abruptly, clients, customers, and employees find themselves talking to new office staff in the centralized location who are less well informed than the previous local office staff. Customers receive incorrect bills, and field employees receive incorrect paychecks.

Difficulties grow as relationships nurtured between the local offices and state agencies are shifted to the anonymous central office. Training of the new employees does not include all of the nuances of each contract that the local offices knew. The personal touch and relationships fostered in the small local office are lost. The contract agencies lose confidence in the new system, and business declines.

An insufficient number of employees are hired to answer the telephones, resulting in unanswered calls. The complex telephone system searches for the next available operator, but customers grow tired of waiting to talk to a real person and turn to other agencies.

Declining business in the pilot site reveals the inadvisability of continuing with the project, and after 5 months the pilot is discontinued. Dismissal of the new employees is inevitable, and shelving of the expensive software is the result. In 2 years the organization is sold to a smaller competitor.

Technology did not fail in this scenario: all of the technology functioned as designed. Lack of money was not the reason for the failure: money was supplied in abundance to try to make this project succeed. Lack of upper management support was not an issue in the failure: upper management firmly supported the concept of automating and centralizing the business. The reasons why this project failed are complex and varied, but one of the major factors was lack of the management of change.

THE IMPACT OF AUTOMATION

When information technology is introduced into an organization, employee behavior changes because the manner of supplying and using information changes. All employees, including professionals, must learn a new way of doing work. Although **managing change** is not specifically an informatics issue, understanding the dynamics of introducing information technology into the system of healthcare delivery is of paramount importance to the success of that installation. According to Simpson (1996), the installation of business-critical systems fails at the rate of about 80 to 90 percent. The failure is not for technological reasons but for behavioral and social reasons. People using the systems are responsible for a majority of the failures.

ORGANIZATIONAL CULTURE

The impact of introducing computer-based information systems in an organization and to its personnel is in part a result of the interaction of such systems with the corporate culture and with the formal and social systems within the organization. **Organizational culture** is a combination of beliefs within the organization about the way work should be organized, the way authority should be exercised, and the way in which people are controlled and rewarded (Handy, 1982). A complex combination of symbols, language, assumptions, and behaviors manifesting themselves in an organization's norms and values make up a culture. Organizational culture is also defined as the pattern of basic assumptions and shared meanings developed by a group to survive its tasks (Schein, 1985), a set of solutions devised by a group to solve common problems (Van Maanen & Barley, 1985), and "the way things are done around here" (Deal & Kennedy, 1982).

According to Smircich (1983), organizational culture serves four functions.

1. It gives a sense of identity to the members.
2. It promotes a sense of commitment to a larger entity.
3. It enhances the stability of the social system.
4. It helps to make sense of behavior. (p. 340)

When an organization introduces computer-based information systems into the work environment, employees are immediately confronted with new artifacts or objects, new technical jargon, and an altered system of beliefs, values, and assumptions about their work lives. Such an enormous change causes a "culture shock," requiring everyone in the organization to adjust to the new way of doing work. Anticipating the adjustment period and managing the change increase the probability of successful system implementation.

The Symbols of Culture

"A culture is dependent upon the nature of the artifacts it uses or the symbols that manifest its ideals" (Romano, 1996, p. 83). The **artifacts** of information system computer workstations include computer manuals, bar coders, automatic medication-dispensing devices, and radio frequency hand-held units. These replace paper charts, kardexes, Post-it notes, clipboards, and forms, the artifacts of a manual system.

Computer technology increases standardization of documentation and introduces new protocols and procedures not previously in place for processing information. Using expert systems to assist the decision-making process directs members of the organization to operate within the guidelines on which the expert system was formulated. Drug-drug interactions and critical results flagging are the earliest examples of this health information technology. Critical paths for medical best practices also guide practitioners to follow a preordained course of care (FitzHenry & Snyder, 1996).

Information system implementation affects the intradepartmental, interdepartmental, and interpersonal communication infrastructures of the organization. Automated documentation may require employees to learn a new standardized language, as discussed in Chapter 5. No longer is narrative, common-language documentation acceptable for gathering information that must be written so that it can be quantified, qualified, trended, queried, and reported. Changing language is often a competence-destroying task for healthcare professionals, who are experts in giving care but novices when learning a new language to describe this care.

Reporting on patients' conditions may be done at a different time and require a different format. A synopsis of patient conditions and care can be generated electronically with a view pertinent to each professional discipline. Decreasing face-to-face reporting can be disconcerting to those who have depended on that mode of communication for giving and receiving information.

Moving patient information from a paper chart in a centralized location to an automated system in a patient's room requires not only learning a new documentation method but also learning how to interact with peers and patients in a new manner. The centralized location of manual charts allows health professionals to examine patient information while socializing and exchanging information with colleagues. This is often done midway through a shift and at the end of a shift. When patient information can be accessed only through computers in the patients' rooms, documentation is done while giving care to each patient and in the presence of the patient rather than colleagues. Terminals are usually placed at the nurses' station as well, but waiting until a more convenient time to document patient information may require jotting notes on a piece of paper as a reminder to create duplicate recordings later. Physicians accustomed to reviewing patient information before entering a patient's room now must do so in the presence of the patient. Not all caregivers are comfortable answering patients' questions while documenting or examining information.

Alterations in the Power Structure

The artifacts of automation may also symbolize shared beliefs of inflexibility, greater control over workers, or reduced inefficiency (Romano, 1996). A computer system allows employees' work to be monitored more closely and for each interaction to be traced back to individual workers. In time, performance evaluations will reflect this process.

Clinical automation alters the **power structure** of the organization by disseminating information to the broader workforce. In a manual information system, the lower on the hierarchy the person, the more dilute the information (Parker et al., 1997). The more senior the management, the more condensed the information. The professional at the point of care seldom sees how his or her individual efforts affect the organization. The accessibility of information in an automated system more easily permits employees to view aggregated and trended information reflecting the status of the organization. The flow of information is also increased through the use of online newsletters, human resources policy manuals, bulletins, and e-mail. Characteristically, highly structured organizational hierarchies tend to discourage communication across departments and projects. Computer-based information systems, however, affect the availability, accessibility, and sharing of information sources at all levels. This, in turn, challenges previous assumptions about internal communication patterns. Centralization or decentralization of decision making may result because of the availability of information to all levels of employees that may change the cultural status quo.

Alterations in Space

The use of space that affects the possible interaction of employees is also affected by the introduction of computer-based information systems. Automation has not met the promise of creating a paperless office. Instead, a deluge of paper has resulted from automation, requiring more space for middle- and lower-level employees. The demands of automation may require the reconceptualization of work and may suggest the need for multiple offices, project rooms, and shared spaces, as well as private work areas (Becker, 1988). The presence of computers also requires the ergonomic considerations that result in changes in seating, lighting, temperature, and noise conditions in the workplace.

Strong cultures either motivate coordinated action and performance or serve as a strong barrier to change (Huber, 1996); therefore, organizational culture becomes an important element to consider when determining how to manage change. Because norms and values are basic and provide comfort, changing cultures is very difficult for all employees.

RESISTANCE TO CHANGE

All organizations resist change (FitzHenry & Snyder, 1996). It has been said that the only person who welcomes change is a wet baby. The initial introduction of automation into a facility is considered a radical change and is the most challenging for managers to facilitate. If the proposed implementation is a modification to an existing system, the change is generally less threatening and somewhat easier to manage (Abbott, 1996). It is safe to assume that every significant health informatics implementation will encounter some resistance; however, the intensity of this resistance can vary widely. In an organization with decent morale and a history of managing changes reasonably well, many employees may be initially neutral toward a particular proposed systems change. However, if previous changes within the organization were poorly managed, employees will avoid involvement because of the negative outcomes of such initiatives in the past.

IMPORTANCE OF MANAGING CHANGE

The introduction of computer-based systems requires a change in the way in which information is acquired, processed, and managed. Because information and its communication is a critical component of organizational culture as well as individual work, changes affecting both must be purposefully managed if the organization is to be effective and the implementation of the information system is to be successful.

The implementation of automated systems brings with it responsibility, opportunity, risk, and change. The change process involves all healthcare professionals as innovators, managers, or recipients of change. Implementation requires intensive planning to prepare users both technically and psychologically. The **psychological aspects** of implementation are process oriented, dealing with the human factors that facilitate or inhibit innovation and change. The **technological preparation** is task oriented, with implementation broken down into step-by-step phases that are focused and manageable. These two processes are not independent of each other, but rather support and undergird each other.

Change processes affect employees' time, energy, and capacities, so managing change in an organization is important for morale and productivity during a difficult time. How an organization manages the change process either impedes or supports the adoption of new behaviors. The pace of change, the resources available for assimilating change, and the procedures in place to implement change need to be examined and understood for their impact on the transfer of learning (Porter-O'Grady & Wilson, 1995).

The **pace of change** in an organization affects the success of the change. Too many changes attempted at one time create a high degree of stress and reduce employees' ability to cope. Large system implementations require a multitude of changes. Perceiving all of the changes as focused on a single ultimate goal enhances employees' ability to cope.

Relevant project management software, standardized implementation guidelines, and change management experts must be readily available during organizational change. Multiple changes can cause information overload, excessive stimulation, distraction from daily operational demands, and burnout in leadership circles. Active strategies to ensure that employees and managers are not robbed of the energy necessary to carry out the changes are mandatory.

Upper management must strongly and publicly support the change initiatives with the human resources, time, and finances necessary to ensure a successful implementation. Those designated as **change managers** must have the time to fulfill their function. The responsibility to direct change cannot be an additional task for managers who already have full-time functions. Without the support of implementation procedures, changes will not be sustained over the long term, will have unanticipated negative outcomes, or will sometimes fail altogether. The result will be distrust of any kind of change.

Management Strategies

Implementation involves working to facilitate the adoption of innovation by planning for and managing change. **Lewin** (1958) describes planned organizational change as a deliberate rather than an inevitable, sudden change that uses strategies to decrease the forces of opposition to change. **Rogers** (1962) defines the adoption of innovation as the decision to continue the use of an idea (which is perceived as new) by the individual.

Change management is the process of assisting individuals and organizations in shifting from an old way to a new way of doing things. Therefore, a change process should both begin and end with a visible acknowledgment or celebration of the impending or just completed change. Other attitudes, environments, or activities necessary to support a change environment are:

- Create an environment in which change is an accepted and expected occurrence.
- Give staff members a vision of the changed environment or system. Focus on how any change will benefit the way people work and improve the outcomes. People want to know how the change affects them and what they do.
- Utilize staff members in planning for the change by providing continuous opportunities to give input.
- Create a plan with staff input regarding the process for the change. Progressively give more people accountability for managing their own change. Changes cannot all occur at one time.
- Determine with staff members how to measure the success of the change.
- Keep communication open and honest.
- Provide ample opportunities for training and education at convenient times and places so that employees are comfortable with the new technology before going "live" with complex functions. People learn by doing. Allow them to practice the new functions, and provide generous support with good information.

- Create a trusting, supportive environment that allows employees to risk failure. Improvisation and experimentation are essential to successful change. Error is a foundation for success.

Effective communication is an essential tool when preparing for change (Abbott, 1996). Unrealistic expectations and miscommunications decrease through effective communication with staff members, practitioners in other disciplines, management, and vendors. Increased awareness of mutual dependence and cooperative partnerships also emerges with increased communication. "The sense of ownership, involvement, and commitment of users can be attained . . . by making the entire process responsive to those it serves" (Abbott, 1996, p. 117).

The home health organization described at the beginning of this chapter violated many of the management strategies listed here. Because of the secret nature of the project, communication was very limited. Employees in the offices had a sense that they would be affected by the new system, but they did not know how. This resulted in great anxiety, built-in resistance to whatever changes would occur, and even sabotage of the information sent to the pilot site. Automating and centralizing all of the operational functions was an overwhelming change, too much to be assimilated at one time. The magnitude of the changes assaulted the organizational culture. The flow of work, authority structures, evaluation mechanisms, employee identity, and geographic location all changed at one time. In addition to lack of communication and changes in the organizational culture, the actual users of the original system were not consulted about their work. This resulted in the deterioration of relationships with referral sources, employees, and clients, causing business to decline. It also caused an underestimation both of the number of telephone calls to be answered and of the complexity of the work. From an understanding of organizational culture and change management, the failure of this expensive project was sadly predictable.

In addition to understanding the organizational culture and the strategies for managing change, an awareness of change theories and strategies is helpful for change managers. Two theorists, Kurt Lewin and Everett Rogers, exemplify an understanding of the behavioral aspects of change and the human decision-making process.

Lewin's Force Field Theory

Perhaps the best known of Kurt Lewin's concepts regarding change is his idea of a "field." Lewin observed that all things happen in what he termed a "force field" (Tiffany & Lutjens, 1998, p. 119). This field consists of social, historical, situational, and physical influences surrounding individuals. Thus Lewin's **force field theory** emphasized relationships between individuals and forces in their environments. Lewin believed that these force fields develop when there is tension within a person. These tensions develop whenever a psychological need or an intention exists, and the tension is released only when the need or intention is fulfilled. The tension may be positive or negative. In force field analysis, change managers identify and analyze the forces in the environment of the individual or group to understand their habits and to discover what to do to change or retain those habits. After analyzing a particular situation, planners will have some idea of what actions will cause change to occur. To make change permanent, strategies must be chosen appropriate to the stage of change involved. According to Lewin (1951), these stages include unfreezing from the present level, moving to the new level, and freezing at the new level (p. 229).

"Unfreezing" is the stage of letting go or realizing that something is lost. It involves softening toward the change and may involve unlearning things that no longer serve the individual's need. This unlearning can create roller-coaster emotions of anxiety, defensiveness, and resistance because it means giving up something familiar and comfortable for something new and often troubling and frustrating. It is a time of separation from the accustomed way of doing things and of changing expectations.

"Moving" is the second stage. This is a transitional stage from the known to the unknown. Loss of control, confusion, negativity, and chaos often characterize this stage as participants seek meaning in the change.

In the third stage, "freezing," new habits or practices become relatively fixed patterns of individual or group functioning. Fear, excitement, enlightenment, or a mixture of these accompanies this stage. Reintegration and recommitment occur at this time. Being cognizant of these steps enables users to anticipate, accept, and act as agents of change rather than products of change (see *Fig. 8.1*).

Rogers's Adopter Categories

Whereas Lewin articulated the process of change, Everett Rogers described the different manners and rates at which individuals respond to innovation or change. Rogers categorized these responses into **adopter**

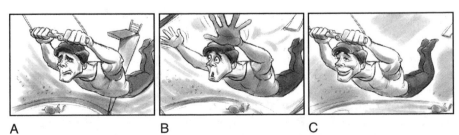

A   B   C

FIGURE 8.1 ▶ Three stages of Lewin's force field theory. (*A*) Unfreezing. (*B*) Moving. (*C*) Freezing.

categories of innovators, early adopters, early majority, late majority, and laggards. Each category consists of individuals with similar degrees of innovativeness. The descriptions of the adopter categories present adopters as ideal types that do not exist in pure form in the real world.

"Innovators" are eager to try new things even before anyone else is aware that something new is available. They are venturesome risk takers who are willing to take a loss. Innovators are not well integrated into the social system but remain on the fringes, as their risk-taking behavior and revolutionary ideas set them apart from their peers. They play an important role in discovering new ideas and introducing them to the local social system, but because they are not a strong part of the peer group, they are not influential in assisting others to adapt to the innovation. They are, however, very useful as members of steering, planning, or equipment committees because of the nature of their personalities (Abbott, 1996). Innovators are too busy looking for the next innovation to assist with the current change process.

"Early adopters" are well integrated into their peer group and are usually the first to accept an innovation. These well-respected people are opinion leaders in their groups, as their judicious selection and early use of an innovation enables them to give what others consider reasoned judgments about the characteristics of the innovation. Their opinion and advice about making decisions to accept or reject a new innovation are sought. Change planners seek early adopters as opinion leaders and role models to guide others toward adopting change.

"Early-majority" individuals adopt new ideas very deliberately: they wait to see how things go with those who adopt earlier. They are willing followers of the early adopters group and therefore play an important role in the change process. Although they are seldom considered to be leaders of opinion, people in this category are great communicators and have many links in important communication networks. Early-majority individuals constitute about one-third of the adopter groups (Tiffany & Lutjens, 1998, p. 221).

"Late-majority" individuals are skeptical about adopting new innovations and usually conform to change as a result of peer pressure, a mandate, or out of economic necessity. This group does not communicate well with others and, as a result, requires intense communication and deliberate facilitation of user involvement. These skeptical persons need abundant evidence to convince them of the desirability and safety of adopting the innovation.

"Laggards" make their adoption decisions last, usually when the next innovation is about to begin. It is only at the time of a new innovation that the laggard will decide that the previous innovation is working fine and he or she does not want to accept the new one. The laggard prefers the past to the future or the present. Members of this group are sometimes considered saboteurs who deliberately undermine the system and encourage others to do the same.

Rogers meant no harm when he used the term "laggard." He wrote that any label applied to the last group to adopt would soon earn a pejorative reputation. He mentioned that the plight of laggards stems not so much from their own characteristics as from social system characteristics that deny them opportunity, creating a precarious economic position for them (Rogers, 1995, pp. 252–280). Determining the source of their resistance and negotiating or modifying the innovation or strategy being used to gain the support and trust of these individuals can positively affect the implementation process.

Change planners are well advised to identify the adopter categories of their change participants, capitalizing on the strengths and attending to the weaknesses of individuals in each category. Innovators are excellent idea generators, but are not helpful with the details and work of implementation. Wise planners will use early adopters, with their energy and opinion-leading characteristics, to chair committees and train others to use the new system. The early majority easily follows the opinion leaders and gives impetus to the change movement. The late majority needs a great deal of information and training to adjust to the innovation. The peer pressure of the early adopters and early majority will help them make the transition to the new way of doing things.

The laggards are not to be ignored. Allowing them to express their fears and concerns through designated channels of communication enables project leaders to examine and address the issues. Spending a great deal of time supporting and coercing the laggards may be a temptation, but greater good will result from investing time in the leaders of the change. Some laggards will never adopt the change and may choose to or be forced to leave. Assessing the characteristics of users assists the change planner in designing strategies to help employees adopt the innovation, manage their time, and focus their energy.

ROLE OF THE HEALTHCARE PROFESSIONAL IN MANAGING CHANGE

Healthcare professionals who understand the importance of managing and processing information to assist with decision making (informatics) are important leaders in managing the innovations that automated systems bring to a work environment. They may not always be involved in the leadership and management of organizational change, but everyone participates in the constantly changing healthcare delivery system and, as such, must assess their own attitudes and actions in regard to change. Whether one is managing the change process or acting as a participant, a primary responsibility in system implementation is influencing others to adopt the innovation. Creating a pro-change environment that readily assimilates new ideas and activities is imperative. Fostering open, honest communication keeps energy focused on problem solving rather than innuendo and rumor. Assuring representation from each professional discipline and user level in discussions about implementation creates an enabling, inclusive atmosphere. Identifying adopter capabilities helps place team members in positions most relevant to their innovation adoption styles. Changes in workflow must begin before final implementation of a new system. To make the transition from manual to automated systems smoother, new documentation methods should be implemented with paper and pencil before they are introduced in automated form. Healthcare professionals may need to help the group learn and accept new values, norms, and assumptions or match a new program to a prior culture.

SUMMARY

The successful implementation of an automated system affects the culture of an organization and requires active management strategies. The innovation may affect, either directly or indirectly, all members of an organizational unit. Change planners need to anticipate the effect of information technology on the operation of the organization, using proactive change management strategies to reduce employee resistance. Knowledge and skillful application of the stages of change and the innovator adopter categories enable the change manager to help employees embrace the new system, ensuring successful use of the new technologies. All healthcare professionals have a role in facilitating group acceptance of the innovation.

▶ LEARNING EXERCISES

1. Describe the culture of your learning institution. How is your work as a student organized? How is authority exercised? How are students controlled and rewarded?
2. How does information technology change the way work is accomplished?
3. How can the implementation of automated systems change authority structures?
4. Brainstorm how the activities of managing change can be carried out.
5. Discuss the stages of unfreezing, moving, and refreezing. Relate the stages to personal change experiences. What were the feelings and actions involved in each stage?
6. What adopter category do you most often belong to in a change situation? How can you identify the categories of others? If you

are the change manager and have identified the adopter categories of your personnel, how would you use that information when planning change management strategies?

7. Discuss various roles for healthcare professionals during times of change.

References

Abbott, P. A. (1996). The nursing manager's role in successful system implementation. In M. E. Mills, C. A. Romano, & B. R. Heller (Eds.), *Information management in nursing and health care* (pp. 117–127). Springhouse, PA: Springhouse.

Becker, F. (1988). Technological innovation and organizational ecology. In M. Helander (Ed.), *Handbook of human–computer interaction* (pp. 1107–1156). New York: Elsevier North-Holland.

Deal, T., & Kennedy, A. (1982). *Corporate culture.* Reading, MA: Addison-Wesley.

FitzHenry, F., & Snyder, J. (1996). Improving organizational processes for gains during implementation. *Computers in Nursing, 14*(3), 171–180.

Handy, C. B. (1982). *Understanding organizations.* Harmonworth, UK: Penguin Books.

Huber, D. (1996). *Leadership and nursing care management.* Philadelphia: W. B. Saunders.

Lewin, K. (1951). Behavior and development as a function of the total situation. In D. Cartwright (Ed.), *Field theory in social science: Selected theoretical papers* (pp. 238–303). Chicago: University of Chicago Press.

Lewin, K. (1958). Group decisions and social change. In E. E. Maccoby, T. M. Newcomb, & E. L. Hartley (Eds.), *Readings in social psychology* (3rd ed., pp. 197–211). New York: Rinehart.

Parker, M., Neimeth, L., & Porter-O'Grady, T. (1997). In T. Porter-O'Grady, M. A. Hawkins, & M. L. Parker (Eds.), *Whole-systems shared governance: Architecture for integration* (pp. 253–288). Gaithersburg, MD: Aspen.

Porter-O'Grady, T., & Wilson, C. K. (1995). *The leadership revolution in health care: Altering systems, changing behaviors.* Gaithersburg, MD: Aspen.

Rogers, E. M. (1962). *Diffusion of innovations.* New York: Free Press.

Rogers, E. M. (1995). *Diffusion of innovations* (4th ed.). New York: Free Press.

Romano, C. A. (1996). Organizational impact of information systems. In M. E. Mills, C. A. Romano, & B. R. Heller (Eds.), *Information management in nursing and health care* (pp. 83–91). Springhouse, PA: Springhouse.

Schein, E. (1985). *Organizational culture and leadership.* San Francisco: Jossey-Bass.

Simpson, R. L. (1996, June). Managing the social and behavioral impact of technology change. *Nursing Management, 27*(6), 26–27.

Smircich, L. (1983). Concepts of culture and organizational analysis. *Administrative Science Quarterly, 28*(3), 339–358.

Tiffany, C. R., & Lutjens, L. R. J. (1998). *Planned change theories for nursing: Review, analysis, and implications.* Thousand Oaks, CA: Sage.

Van Maanen, J., & Barley, S. (1985). Cultural organization: Fragments of a theory. In P. Frost, L. Moore, M. Louis, C. Lundberg, & J. Martin (Eds.), *Organizational culture* (pp. 31–53). Beverly Hills, CA: Sage.

9

Information Systems Cycle

LEARNING OBJECTIVES

By the end of this chapter, you will be able to:
❱ Describe the four parts of the system cycle
❱ Identify the most important element of the system cycle
❱ Describe how the focus of system implementation has changed over time
❱ List the steps in each phase of the system cycle
❱ Describe the types of benefits that may be achieved with the implementation of a new system
❱ List reasons for implementation failures

In the novel and film *Field of Dreams,* an Iowa farmer plows under a field of corn and builds a complete baseball field because voices whisper to him, "If you build it, they will come." In the story, a dream team of baseball legends does come and play, justifying the farmer's seemingly senseless actions.

New interactive technologies are also seductive. The lure of the hardware, the flash of "look what we can do," leads organizations to ill-considered and ultimately useless system development. Sometimes it seems as though the developers hear voices saying, "If you build it, they will use it," and they pursue system construction with little regard for the user or the outcomes. Such systems produce glitzy programs with bells and whistles that may not be used or, if used, may not accomplish anything useful.

THE OXFORD INCIDENT

The "Oxford incident" involved a company that rose on the basis of its own innovations, including the automation of systems, and ultimately was buried by them. By the fall of 1997, Oxford Health Plans of Norwalk, Connecticut, was the largest health maintenance organization (HMO) in the state of New York and one of the fastest growing in the country, with 1.9 million members (Schriner, 1998). It enjoyed a nationwide reputation for innovation and cost-effective actions. For 5 years the company had struggled to create new information systems to handle the growth. According to Schriner (1998), the new systems failed miserably: customers were not billed for premiums, and providers went unpaid for months. Oxford wrote off uncollectable revenues and advanced payment to providers without knowing the real costs. On October 24, 1997, the company made public third-quarter losses of $78 million. Wall Street cashed out, and Oxford's stock fell from $62 to $25 in a single day. Fourth-quarter losses added up to $120 million or more in estimated losses, causing Oxford's stock to drop even lower.

According to Thomas Johnson, a healthcare consultant with Sheldon I. Dorenfest Associates in Chicago, Oxford's managers were ahead of their time. "They had great product ideas. They had great market ideas that were very innovative. But then they didn't manage the process" (Schriner, 1998, p. 86). What was unmanaged was not only the change process but also the process of implementing a new system. Oxford Health Plans tried to create its own information system, but the programmers could not keep pace with the company's needs, and managers wanted the systems to do more than they were capable of doing. Without proper management of the cycle of system implementation, the company faltered and fell.

HISTORY OF THE SYSTEMS IMPLEMENTATION FOCUS

Systems planning and implementation are based not only on the capabilities of information technology but also on forces in the environment that affect health care. According to Jenkins (1995), healthcare computer decisions in the 1970s were primarily financially oriented. Consequently, the patient billing process, the general ledger, and accounts payable were automated. Often the systems were created and programmed within the organization.

In the 1980s, the emphasis on automation broadened to focus on ancillary systems such as laboratory, pharmacy, and radiology systems. Software vendors created niche markets specializing in a single area in which they were proficient. Many of these vendors created stand-alone, self-contained systems that were not integrated with other systems. Information could not be shared among departments. The radiology department, the laboratory, and the admitting department each entered its own patient information. Each system duplicated the other for patient information.

In the 1990s, the trend became documentation of patient care at the bedside. Vendors concentrated on broad-based, integrated systems in which information flowed easily from one department to the other, without duplicate and redundant entry, solving the problems of the previous decade. However, broad-based systems cannot always address all of the intricacies of specialized areas. Niche market vendors concentrating in one area generally meet the needs of that area with greater attention to detail.

In the future, system implementation will have greater emphasis on niche market vendors who can interface their programs with the programs of other vendors, creating seamless delivery of information across departments. Creating partnerships among large, broad-based information technology vendors and small, niche market vendors solves the problem of integration while meeting the information needs of specialty areas.

THE INFORMATION SYSTEMS CYCLE

The desire for greater cost effectiveness and better-quality healthcare, the push toward integrated healthcare delivery systems and community care networks, the growth of managed care and capitation, and the increase in mergers, acquisitions, and other forms of collaboration among healthcare providers place additional burdens on existing healthcare information systems, as well as heightening the expectations of what information systems can achieve in the future. By knowing what current automated systems can achieve, and by learning the steps necessary to reap more of the potential benefits of clinical information systems, healthcare organizations can gain greater efficiency, better patient care, and a greater return on information systems programs (Dorenfest, 1997). Advances in information technology improve access to healthcare information, operational efficiency, and clinical effectiveness. To ensure appropriate use of technology and information systems, careful planning, selection, implementation, and maintenance are mandatory.

The four stages of software and hardware selection are known as the "systems cycle" *(Fig. 9.1)*. The stages are:

- **Analysis**
- **Design**
- **Development**
- **Implementation**

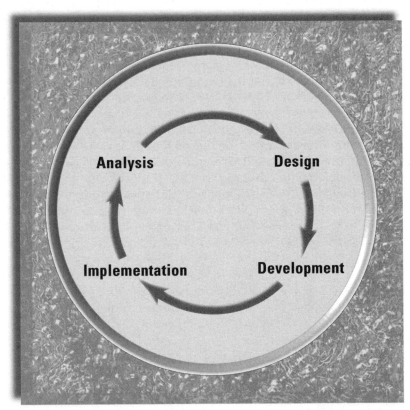

FIGURE 9.1 ▶ Systems cycle.

The last stage, implementation, includes ongoing evaluation. Evaluation generally leads to identification of further efficiencies to be achieved, initiating the analysis phase again and perpetuating the cycle.

ANALYSIS

The first phase of the system cycle, analysis, includes **definition of the problem, analysis of benefits,** creation of a **project definition document,** allocation of **resources, request for information** and **request for proposal,** identification of short list, site visits, identification of two finalists, and negotiation of the contract *(Box 9.1)*. Analysis is the most important step in the system cycle, as it identifies the purpose of the implementation and outlines the expectations of the project. Without problem identification or enhancement definition, design and development remain unfocused and evaluation is unmeasurable.

Definition of the Problem

Analysis begins by identifying a problem or inefficiency that requires a solution and then determining the best solution. Organizations often neglect this step, dazzled by a sales presentation touting the wonders of an automated system. Carried away by the enthusiasm of the presenter, the organization then tries to find a problem that the automated system can solve. Only by thorough identification of a problem and exploration of a variety of solutions (that may not even include automation) can the organization determine that automation will bring benefits.

Informatics, when focused on building healthcare systems that will be routinely used, should be problem driven. Informatics should be concerned, first and foremost, with understanding the nature of information and communication problems in healthcare. Only then should informat-

---

BOX 9.1   ANALYSIS PHASE OF THE SYSTEMS CYCLE

- Define the problem
- Analyze the benefits
- Determine the project definition document
- Allocate resources
- Write specifications
- Send the RFI and RFP
- Identify vendors on the short list
- Visit sites
- Identify two finalists
- Negotiate the contract

ics try to determine if it is appropriate for technology to solve these problems and, if necessary, develop and apply these technologies (Coiera, 1997, p. 75).

Benefits Analysis

Identification of a problem or inefficiency requires a determination of benefits. Benefits are expected, potential, or realized. An **expected benefit** is identified as "an outcome that the healthcare facility identifies as important to its clinical and business needs, anticipates achieving and actively pursues" (Hoehn, 1996, p. 100). If the problem is that too much time is required for quality assurance (QA) reviews, then an expected benefit resulting from the solution is reduced time required for QA reviews. A **potential benefit** is "any improvement or positive outcome that is possible or likely to occur through the implementation of a clinical information system" (Hoehn, 1996, p. 100). A potential benefit of automating the electronic health record may include greater accuracy while performing QA reviews. A **realized benefit** is a "positive outcome or improvement in clinical or business operations that has actually already occurred. It may be an actively pursued benefit or one that is inherent in the implementation of the new system" (Hoehn, 1996, p. 100). A realized benefit of an electronic health record shows that QA takes 1 hour per chart with the manual system but takes 15 minutes with the automated system. The realized benefit is 45 minutes of saved time.

All too often, new systems are implemented with a *Field of Dreams* mentality, meaning that with the introduction of an automated system, benefits will occur. However, not articulating the expected and potential benefits at the onset of the project eliminates the possibility of measuring the benefits realized at the end of the implementation. A proactive approach must be used to identify potential and expected benefits, establish a plan for achieving the benefits, and develop a method for establishing a baseline and tracking the results against the plan.

Whenever possible, expected benefits should be quantifiable by stating the benefits in measurable terms. Some benefits are not quantifiable but only qualifiable. They are subjective, such as client and employee satisfaction. Decreasing the error rate is measurable, but the reduction in human suffering achieved by decreasing the error rate is very difficult to measure. Efforts must be made to determine both quantifiable and qualifiable benefits.

Process Improvement

Healthcare systems often spend thousands, even millions, of dollars on technology, only to find that many operational problems still exist and new problems often develop. The reason for the failure of an information system to live up to its promise is that the organization did not first examine the processes automated. Simply automating existing workflow processes does not guarantee success. Evaluation of current workflow to determine the need for change before automation begins is critical. Virtually all of the activities within healthcare are processes, and it is these processes, not departments, that run the healthcare organization (Dorenfest, 1997). **Process improvement** activities should focus on the whole process rather than on individual departments, should address the interdisciplinary nature of the process, and should result in simplification, not increased confusion *(Box 9.2)*. The purpose of process improvement is to simplify the processes through redesign to eliminate possible bottlenecks and obstacles. Human factors analysis is fundamental in the evaluation of processes. While technology can significantly improve effi-

---

BOX 9.2   EXAMPLE OF AN INTERDEPARTMENTAL PROCESS

A simple laboratory order may contain these elements:

- Physician writes order
- Unit clerk transcribes it onto an order form or enters it into the computer, triggering the specimen collection process
- Nurse or technician gets specimen from patient
- Specimen transported to laboratory, triggering the laboratory order fulfillment process and the billing process
- Laboratory does many fulfillment steps, such as:
  Scheduling the test
  Updating the status and making it available to nurses and other clinicians
  Conducting the test
  Posting and distributing the results (paper or electronic)
- Some billing steps include:
  Posting line item detail to account
  Determining amount due by guarantor, payer, etc.
  Preparing the bill at discharge or at the scheduled interim time
  Reviewing and sending the bill
  Collecting payment
- Nurse views results
- Physician views results
- Results posted to patient chart (part of medical records/charting process)

Adapted from Dorenfest, 1997.

ciency and help reduce costs, its full benefits can be realized only when efficient and effective work processes are already in place. Improving processes before implementing an automated information system enables quicker implementation, often at a lower cost, as well as reaping real operational savings (Maguire & Frohwerk, 1998).

Project Definition

Professionals from all of the healthcare disciplines play a pivotal role in developing sound selection and implementation strategies. Today's movement toward multidisciplinary, patient-centered care requires all clinical disciplines as well as technical support individuals to be involved in clinical information system selection. After identification of the problem, articulation of the expected and potential benefits, and analysis of the present processes, the multidisciplinary team can create a project definition document.

A written project definition document includes answers to the following questions:

- What is the real problem to be solved and/or stated goals to be realized?
- Why accomplish the project?
- What are specific outcomes expected from the project?
- What is to be accomplished in the project?
- What are the measurable benefits from the above outcomes?
- What are the estimated costs?
- What is the justification for the project, including the relationship between costs and benefits?
- What are the assumptions that support the project?
- What are the known constraints on the project?
- What are the boundaries/limitations of the project?
- What are the project risks and their causes?
- What is the timing of the remaining phases of the project?
- Who will be committed to implementing the project, and what positions do they hold?

—Saba & McCormick, 1996, p. 272.

Allocating Resources

The project definition document assists with identification of human resources required for the remainder of the analysis phase. Contrary to what often happens, which is adding analysis responsibilities to an employee's already full workload, individuals must be identified to do the analysis and given the time to complete the work. In addition to human resources, finances and facilities for the work must be firmly committed before the process can fulfill its stated objectives.

Request for Information/Proposal

After looking at existing systems within the organization, the task force assigned to the analysis phase can develop criteria for its vision of the ideal system and send a **request for information** (RFI) to as many vendors as possible. An RFI provides some general information about the institution and requests a general response from the vendors regarding the types of products they manufacture and market.

Developing a **request for proposal** (RFP) is the next step. An RFP is much more detailed than an RFI and includes a formal statement describing the organization, its objectives, functional requirements for an automated system, budgetary constraints, and schedules. Vendors are given a time frame, usually 30 days, in which to respond about their ability to meet the specifications. No one vendor meets all the needs of the organization. The organization must determine what functions are necessary, what functions are desirable, and what functions are nice to have. These determinations assist both the vendor's evaluation of its ability to meet the specifications and the organization's determination of the vendor's ability to provide the desired product.

At the conclusion of the RFP time period, the task force evaluates the responses. An evaluation matrix helps score the vendor's ability to fulfill the system's requirements. Ranking the evaluation scores identifies the top three or four vendors meeting the system's requirements. This is referred to as the "short list" of vendors competing for the sale.

Site Visits

The next phase of the evaluation usually involves visits to locations where computer systems similar to the one proposed by the vendor are installed and operational. The purpose of site visits is to inspect the systems under consideration. It is important to choose a site that matches the facility's size and organizational culture. Before the visit, the site visit team develops criteria, questions, and an agenda for the host to follow *(Box 9.3)*. It is important that the site visit team include members of the task force as well as end users of the system. Schedule as much time as possible with the end users at the host site and ask to have site representatives in similar positions available. For instance, a respiratory therapist or an intensive care unit (ICU) nurse from the host site should be available to talk to his or her visiting counterpart.

Final Choice

Using the information from the site visits, choose two vendors who demonstrate the ability to fulfill the system's requirements. Senior manage-

---

Box 9.3   SITE VISIT QUESTIONS

- Is the product easy to use?
- Does the system meet regulatory agency requirements?
- Does the facility have any interfaces, and how do they work?
- Has the facility experienced any unplanned downtime?
- How responsive is the vendor to problems?
- How good was vendor support during implementation?
- What is the satisfaction level of end users since implementation?
- Does the response time meet the needs of the users?
- Have any benefits been demonstrated since the system was implemented?
- What security measures are in place?
- Has the facility participated in any product users' groups? If so, were they beneficial?
- What reports are generated?
- Can ad hoc reports be written, and are examples available?
- Does the facility have confidence in the vendor?

Adapted from Malinowski and Potter, 1997.

---

ment contacts the preferred vendor and the second choice. Contract negotiations take place between the organization and the vendors of choice. After the negotiations, choose one vendor to develop the system.

DESIGN PHASE

The second phase, design, begins after purchasing the system. This phase includes benefits management, resource allocation, development of a time frame, cost/budget analysis, determination of facilities and equipment, design of input and output criteria, screen flow design, interfaces, workflow assessment, and determination of controls for data security, warnings, and reminders (Box 9.4). The continued involvement of a multidisciplinary team is vital to the success of the process.

Benefits Management

Establishing a **benefits management plan** involves identifying the expected and potential benefits of the system and measuring the present processes. If the nursing department is implementing a documentation system that includes care planning, and the expected benefit is greater accuracy and decreased time in writing care plans, documenting and measuring the present care-planning process is a must. Measurements

Box 9.4   Design Phase

- Plan benefits management
- Allocate resources
- Develop time frame
- Perform cost/budget analysis
- Determine facilities and equipment
- Design input/output criteria
- Design screen flows
- Determine workflow
- Determine controls for warnings and reminders

may include the length of time taken to complete an individualized care plan on a new admission, the adequacy of the plan, and determination of the relationship between the plan of care and the actual care given to the patient on a daily basis. These same measurements take place after the new system is implemented and the learning curve levels out. Employees learning new systems require a period of time to flatten the learning curve, accept the new process, and utilize the new automated system appropriately and effectively. An adequate amount of time should pass before determining the realization of any benefits. Comparison of the "before" and "after" measurements determines the realized benefits.

Resource Allocation

As in the analysis phase, allocating resources is necessary to see the project through to completion. The project staff appointed at the beginning of the investigation should, if possible, be retained for the duration of the project. All disciplines and departments affected by the implementation and the technical information systems department must be represented on the team. Clinical personnel with an understanding of automated systems who are on the team act as a liaison between the end users and the programmers. A systems manager may be selected from any department, but he or she must be a capable administrator. Such a person not only supervises the development of the system but also administers project staff personnel, time, budget control, and cost activities.

Time Frame

A time frame for outlining and synchronizing all the steps in developing the information system moves the project along in a timely fashion. Several project management tools can help control and report the status of the project. They include a Gantt chart, which identifies tasks over time, and a PERT chart system, which identifies critical dependencies among tasks (Jaworski, 1997, p. 122). Although the time frame requires adjustment periodically, it provides a date-driven goal and a method of measuring how well the project is proceeding.

Cost/Budget Analysis

Performing a **cost/budget analysis** to implement information technology occurs early in the project. Some costs, such as hardware and software costs, are obvious, but organizations must not be caught by the "iceberg effect" *(Fig. 9.2)*. Just as the bulk of an iceberg is hidden below the surface of the water, substantial costs in an implementation project are also often hidden below the surface. Costs that are not readily apparent, but that must be considered, are service contracts, upgrades, interfaces, initial and ongoing training, evaluation, and increased technical personnel.

Facilities and Equipment

Automated systems require hardware, software, and peripheral equipment. Making decisions about client server technology, mainframes, large minicomputer systems, and other storage systems such as optical

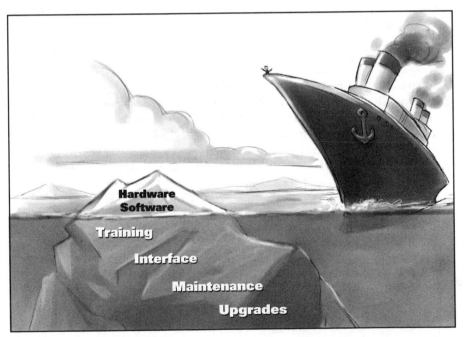

FIGURE 9.2 ▶ Iceberg effect.

imaging systems is essential. All of the equipment must be purchased and properly housed. At this time, preliminary decisions are made about the amount and placement of hardware for individual units. Considerations include whether to have desktop, bedside, and/or wireless technology. Planning begins for workstation space, placement for wall-mounted devices, carts for portable devices, and the electrical supply for hardware, including printers. Preliminary planning also considers the environmental factors of noise, lighting, activity level, and ergonomics. Facility activities require planning office space for an increasing number of technical support staff and training rooms.

Input and Output Designs

Designing the **inputs** is a major step in system design (Saba & McCormick, 1996, p. 281). Inputs (data) are entered into fields to create records that in turn make up databases. Inputs determine **outputs**. If data are never entered, they can never be retrieved. The content of each input must be specified in detail to meet output requirements. The most definable elements are used as inputs; for example, the birth date but not the age of a patient should be entered as an input. Frequently used data, such as the patient's name and allergies, must be gathered only once and then designed to appear where necessary in screen flow. Manual forms used before automation provide a reference for data that are necessary for information management. Details of alphanumeric content, number of digits or letters, documentation format, specialized language, and any required calculations are important to input design.

Designing outputs is concurrent with or even precedes the design of inputs. If data are gathered but never used as output, data can be eliminated. The design of outputs specifies the form of the output, such as a report, graph, chart, or table. In system design, detailed descriptions of the content, format, medium, estimated volume, frequency, and distribution of output are essential.

Screen Flow Design

The content of each screen requires thoughtful design. One of the great advantages of paper is that it demands little structuring. The recording of data on paper is unconstrained in both form and content. A manual record accommodates a physical examination with hand-drawn diagrams or a long, detailed narrative containing subjective assessments of a patient's mental state. When redesigning the flow of information for an automated form, the constraints of automation must be considered in the design. Both the flexibility to accommodate a variety of presentations and enough structure to reduce errors that may occur from the omission of data are necessary for **screen flow** design.

Flexibility in moving from one screen to another is also a screen design consideration. If a potential client for home health services calls, the data-gathering screens for client intake must be flexible enough to move quickly from one topic to another. Although the sequence of the flow of information is anticipated, clients do not always give information in the anticipated order. The intake coordinator may want to start the intake process with demographic information, but the client may want to give medical history information. Flexibility in screen design enables the user to move quickly from one area to another while providing **reminders** about gathering essential information. The screens must be flexible enough to receive information in a variety of arrangements.

Screen flow designers need to know the sequence of anticipated data entry. Entry of vital signs normally occurs in the order of temperature, pulse, and respiration. To change that order when designing a screen invites error. The end user must be actively involved in the design of the screen flow.

The iterative process of beginning by designing screens on paper and moving to actually programming screens is the most cost- and time-effective method of design. Presenting paper screens representing actual screens to the users solicits feedback, which is used to adjust the design. Paper screens are quickly and easily modified. After the users accept them, the more expensive programming can begin.

Interfaces

When designing a system, the most important thing to bear in mind is the ability to share information. Applications purchased from different vendors usually will not share information without specific programming that allows each application to **interface** or share information with the others. For instance, information from a hospital admitting system purchased from one vendor may not flow to an application scheduling patients for the operating room (OR) purchased from another vendor. Patient demographic information, diagnosis, allergies, room number, and physician information captured during the admission process will not appear on the OR scheduling screen without an interface. If creating an interface is not possible, all patient information must be reentered. Since creating an interface is not always possible, it is important to consider the need for and the ability to create interfaces when investigating the purchase of systems. Each vendor involved in the interface must supply interface programming. Programming interfaces is costly and is part of the cost and budgeting considerations.

Workflow

Planning for a change in process and **workflow** should be addressed and implemented during the design phase. The transition to a new system is less traumatic if a change in policy and procedures across all involved units/departments is phased into normal activities before switching to the automated system. For example, if the method of ordering laboratory tests changes drastically with the implementation of the new system, modeling and standardizing the new method is necessary during the design phase. Plan to document, distribute, and incorporate the new method into normal operating procedures long before the transition to the new system.

Controls

The design of controls ensures that input data are correctly processed, output information is complete and accurate, and no data have been lost or stolen (Saba & McCormick, 1996, p. 283). The system's ability to process information from input to output is audited to determine accuracy and reduce system errors.

Another type of control involves development of a plan for backup files. Backup files are generally stored off site to protect the data in the event of a natural disaster at the primary site. System controls protect the security and safety of the data files. Identifying procedures to protect the confidentiality of patient information in an electronic system is a requisite. Another necessity to address is employee confidentiality agreements with electronic data and multiple access sites in mind.

Controls are also designed for data fields. If a Social Security number is always a nine-digit number, then it is essential to program the field receiving that data to accept only nine digits. Decisions about mandatory and nonmandatory fields affect screen flow design and data integrity. Patient name is an example of a mandatory field. Without the patient name, even if the name is "John Doe," the other patient information is useless.

DEVELOPMENT

During the development phase, the designs finalized during the previous phase are enhanced, modified, built, and tested. The development phase includes determining standardization and uniqueness, building data files, testing the system, and developing supporting documents (Box 9.5). The development phase does not have a large number of steps but may take a long time, depending on the size of the files requiring data entry.

Box 9.5   Development Phase

- Determine standardization/uniqueness
- Build data files
- Test
- Develop support documents

Determining Standardization and Uniqueness

As much of the system as possible should be standardized. When designs deviate from a standard and are customized, costs increase, development time lengthens, and implementation work for future upgrades increases in both time and cost. Although standardization for all units and disciplines may be ideal, it is not always practical. An ICU uses different terminology, looks at information in a different manner, and uses equipment different from that of an ambulatory clinic. A respiratory therapist has different documentation requirements than a cardiac technician.

Groups of end users must closely examine their automation needs to determine the extent of customization required to support their practice. Units that have previously considered themselves unique may realize that they can standardize more than they anticipated. Teamwork is an essential component of the customization/standardization stage. Implementation team members are the conduits between their unit and the team. Communication with the end users on various units is important in both the development of the system and the acceptance of the cultural change the implementation brings.

Building Data Files

After any customization is determined, building of the data files can begin. The first step is entering the inputs designed during the previous phase into the system. Vendors may provide a template to add or delete information. Patient historical files may require entry. Laboratory values, standardized care plans, and the hospital formulary must be built so that the information can be drawn on.

Dedicating personnel to data entry speeds up the process. End users or data entry personnel can build the files. End users have the ability to solve any problems about entering the information because they understand how the information will be used. Data entry personnel may be faster at the actual entry process. At times, the volume of information to be entered is so great that several months are required to complete the process.

Testing the System

After the files are built, the system is tested to ensure that all data are processed correctly and to generate the desired outputs. **System testing** occurs in two phases, system testing and acceptance testing. A professional team representing the vendor performs system testing, and the users perform acceptance testing. Once system testing is completed, acceptance testing begins. Each unit and discipline helps the system analysts design test plans for validation. Test plans allow for the testing of application software and ultimately determine if the systems function in an integrated mode. This critical stage of testing determines if the system functions according to the specifications developed in the analysis phase. In system testing, individual modules are tested independently and then tested as part of an integrated system. Scenarios incorporated into test plans must be clinically realistic, and testing must take many variables into account. These variables include entering data correctly into the system to verify appropriate components of the system and entering erroneous data into the system in order to validate the interaction of tables and files within the system, as identified by specific departments (Glacey et al., 1990). Particular attention should be paid to the interface between programs, especially with the transfer of data between modules/departments. Output should be validated, and the flow of data must be tracked (Abbott, 1996, p. 123).

Developing Documentation

Developing **documentation** is an ongoing activity involving both the vendor and the purchasing organization. Vendors provide documentation of the operating system describing what data are input, their processing procedure, and the way in which particular outputs are generated, as well as maintenance manuals detailing how the system is maintained, updated, and repaired. Operator guides include flow charts, program specifications, backup and recovery procedures, table and record layouts, operational procedures, and a dictionary of terms (Abbott, 1996, p. 123).

The vendor may supply user manuals discussing how to use the system, but more often the purchasing organization creates them as it integrates automated processes with regular operating procedures of the institution. User manuals are nontechnical, step-by-step instructions for each process involving an end user. Conveniently locating user manuals in work areas increases accessibility for users.

IMPLEMENTATION

The last phase of the system cycle is implementation of the system. The implementation phase includes training, final testing, conversion to the new system, and postimplementation evaluation *(Box 9.6)*.

BOX 9.6   IMPLEMENTATION PHASE

- Train users
- Perform final testing
- Convert to new system
- Evaluate the process

Training

The training step is not the first time the end users hear about the system. According to Abbott (1996, p. 122), education precedes training and "clarifies the strategic information services plan, unfreezes attitudes, heightens awareness of mission and organizational objectives, and assists learners in understanding the impact of the system on work practices. Education also serves to lessen resistance, encourage user acceptance, and foster true involvement."

Training familiarizes end users with the specifics of the system as it relates to their activities. It is essential that users learn to use the system properly and with a minimum of frustration. Unit managers choose employees who learn to be expert users and trainers. Early adopters make excellent expert users, as they are eager to adopt the new system and are already looked on as role models by other employees. These expert users will then train others on their unit, and are available after implementation for support and system problem solving. The vendor provides train-the-trainer sessions to the small group who become the expert users.

Training is resource intensive, and requires planning and coordination among trainers and managers. The majority of healthcare organizations operate 24 hours a day, 7 days a week, so training must be available at the times convenient for the staff. Decisions on scheduling classes during working time or outside normal working hours affect employee compliance. Retention of information is greatest when short training sessions are held as close to the conversion date as possible (Denger et al., 1988). Training of personnel depends on the type and amount of interaction they have with the new system. Those heavily involved with the system require more in-depth training than those who use the system just for data entry. Depending on the size of the training room facilities, instruction ranges from large groups to one-on-one tutoring. Training generally consists of a combination of an overview discussion, demonstration of the system, and hands-on practice. The user manual provides the supporting documentation for training and acts as a reference for the students.

Final Testing

Final testing of the system involves running parallel systems, both manual and automated, at the same time. User involvement adds reality to the real-time simulations. The integrity of the data input is compared to that of the data output, timeliness of the transactions is monitored, and comprehensiveness of the procedures is evaluated. If the parallel testing is successful, selecting a conversion date is the next step.

Conversion

Conversion is the process of replacing the old system with the new one and is often referred to as "going live." The conversion process can take many forms, and the form chosen dictates how the process will actually take place. Go-live methods include parallel, phased, pilot, and big bang. Advantages and disadvantages exist for each method, and no one method can be used in all situations.

The parallel approach is a conservative, safe method of conversion, but it requires duplicate work and is expensive. The parallel approach runs the old and new systems side by side for a period of time. The old system supports the business of the work while the new system runs in a test mode. Slowly the new system takes over all processing, and the old system becomes a backup and verification. Once everyone is completely satisfied with the new system, the old system is removed.

The phased approach compartmentalizes the new system into modules. Modules are introduced one at a time. When one module is operating satisfactorily, the next module is introduced. Training for this method is complicated, as users must be trained on one module at a time. Alternatively, if training includes all the modules, communication about the introduction schedule must be intense.

The pilot method introduces the entire system to one unit at a time. The first unit in the pilot method determines if the system is functioning appropriately and if the users are receiving adequate training. During the pilot unit session, the final bugs in the system are eliminated and any training weaknesses are corrected before the next unit goes live.

The big bang approach involves switching from one system to another all at once. This method may be the most risky, but some circumstances require it. An advantage of this method is that it shortens the period of organizational anxiety. Also, personnel who provide support for more than one unit are provided with continuity of the system. Disadvantages include less control of the implementation and the need for greater support.

The go-live process is the most intense step in the system cycle. It requires 24-hour coverage by the implementation team for the first few days, with around-the-clock support for the following few weeks. The information services department must provide an immediate response to technical problems during this period.

Evaluation

Evaluating the system is the final step in the implementation process. This step is often minimized or totally ignored. The postimplementation evaluation assesses whether the stated objectives of the system have been achieved. A **system evaluation** involves comparing a working system with its requirements to determine how well the requirements are met, to determine the possibilities for growth and improvement, and to preserve the lessons of a computerization project in preparation for future efforts (Saba & McCormick, 1996, p. 291). The benefits management plan from the design phase is carried for 6 months to 2 years after implementation by measuring in the new system the same processes used in the old system. The comparison of the measurements determines if the expected benefits have been realized. Potential benefits are also investigated. Sharing the benefits achieved assists personnel during the refreezing stage in the change process. The lessons learned in the evaluation of one implementation are used to increase the efficiency and effectiveness of the next implementation or upgrade.

WHY SOME PROJECTS FAIL

Because projects do fail, planning for failures must be part of system management. Understanding why projects fail can facilitate the procurement and management of systems that handle failures gracefully and safely and minimize interruptions to workflow. Projects fail for a number of reasons. Some of the most common reasons are:

- Lack of a clearly defined and documented vision
- Inadequate or inappropriate resources
- Lack of planning
- Lack of training
- Hardware failure
- Software failure
- Failure to maintain equipment
- Inadequate testing
- Unrealistic expectations

According to Jaworski (1997, p. 123), the key to success is to define the project's scope and expectations clearly, plan to meet those expectations, and establish a change control process. Change control, risk management, and issues management help ensure clear documentation, accuracy of the project's scope, and analysis in terms of impact and approval.

SUMMARY

This chapter has outlined the four phases of the systems cycle: analysis, design, development, and implementation. The most important phase of the cycle is analysis. Without a complete understanding of the problems to be overcome or the processes to be enhanced, there is no blueprint to guide the design and development of the system. No evaluation can take place without identification of the benefits to be achieved. A well-constructed analysis defines the evaluation process. Evaluation clarifies the strengths and weaknesses of the system, paving the way for the next analysis, thereby starting the cycle again.

Automation continues to pervade the healthcare delivery system, creating a constant need to implement and upgrade automated systems. All healthcare professionals will be involved at some point in the system cycles of the future. Professionals knowledgeable about the system cycle process are a valuable asset to their organization.

▶ LEARNING EXERCISES

1. Discussion questions:
   - Why is analysis the most important step? What happens if this step is neglected?
   - Are all the components of the systems cycle necessary for every type of implementation—for instance, an ICU monitoring system?
   - What is the role of each discipline during the systems cycle?
   - How do different types of implementation affect different disciplines?
2. Name factors that may be part of the iceberg effect.
3. Create an outpatient, public health, clinic, or ambulatory care systems cycle scenario. Discuss any differences noted from the acute care implementation.
4. Compare the systems cycle outlined in this volume with the systems cycle described in another volume. How are they the same? How do they differ?
5. List the human factors considerations relevant to the design and development phases.

References

Abbott, P. A. (1996). The nursing manager's role in successful system implementation. In M. E. C. Mills, C. A. Romano, & B. R. Heller (Eds.), *Information management in nursing and health care* (pp. 117–127). Springhouse, PA: Springhouse.

Coiera, E. (1997). *Guide to medical informatics, the Internet and telemedicine.* London: Chapman & Hall.

Denger, S., Cole, D., & Walker, H. (1988). Implementing an integrated clinical information system. *Journal of Nursing Administration, 18*(12), 28–34.

Dorenfest, S. I. (1997). Emerging trends in health care information systems: Increasing focus on process improvement benefits through clinical automation. *Proceedings of the annual Healthcare Information and Management Systems Society (HIMSS) conference, 1,* 453–460. Chicago: HIMSS.

Glacey, T. S., Brooks, G. M., & Vaughan, V. S. (1990, March/April). Hospital information systems. *Computers in Nursing, 8*(2), 55–59.

Hoehn, B. J. (1996). Benefits management. In M. E. C. Mills, C. A. Romano, & B. R. Heller (Eds.), *Information management in nursing and health care* (pp. 99–107). Springhouse, PA: Springhouse.

Jaworski, M. A. (1997). Project management. In N. A. Kreider & B. J. Hazelton (Eds.), *The systems challenge* (pp. 113–127). Chicago: American Hospital Association.

Jenkins, S. (1995). Nurses' responsibilities in the implementation of information systems. In M. J. Ball, K. J. Hannah, S. K. Newbold, & J. V. Douglas (Eds.), *Nursing informatics.* New York: Springer-Verlag.

Maguire, L., & Frohwerk, A. (1998, July). Process first, technology second. *Healthcare Informatics, 76.*

Malinowski, A., & Potter, L. (1997). Selection of hardware and software. In N. A. Kreider & B. J. Haselton (Eds.), *The systems challenge* (pp. 129–146). Chicago: Americal Hospital Association.

Saba, V. A., & McCormick, K. A. (1996). *Essentials of computers for nurses* (2nd ed). New York: McGraw-Hill.

Schriner, M. W. (1998, February). Oxfordphobia. *Healthcare Informatics,* 85–92.

10 Information for Managing Health

LEARNING OBJECTIVES

By the end of this chapter, you will be able to:
▶ Discuss the historical background leading to managed care
▶ Define managed care

▶ Assess the advantages and disadvantages of managed care
▶ Describe codes and measurements used in managing care
▶ Discuss the role of information in managing health
▶ Describe the role of allied health professionals in managing health

In the early 1990s, the state of Virginia's Medicaid office watched emergency department visits plummet 39 percent for a group of asthmatics enrolled in a pilot disease management program. Despite increased use of more expensive corticosteroids, its $200,000 investment realized a $3 million savings in the first year, says Steven Sutor, president of Adventa Health Education, Baltimore (Marietti, 1999). By avoiding many of the usual high-cost crisis interventions and using a bottom-up clinical approach to disease management, Virginia's Medicaid program got a 15-fold return on investment by training physicians in basic communication skills and best practices and by bringing patients into an organized care management program.

Containing the cost of healthcare by managing an individual's health is the hallmark of the healthcare delivery system of the 1990s and the twenty-first century. As this new driving force of healthcare delivery evolves, it evokes strong emotions in both providers and consumers. Both feel a loss of decision-making autonomy to a system over which they believe they have no control. Control of decisions about healthcare delivery increasingly lies in the quality, management, and processing of information in managed care systems such as **health maintenance organizations (HMOs)**.

HMOs are not a new phenomenon. The oldest HMO is Kaiser Permanente, established in 1945 to help the industrialist Henry Kaiser provide healthcare to his shipbuilding employees (Schneider, 1998). However, it is only recently that the HMO concept has really grown. Since 1990, the number of Americans enrolled in HMOs has increased 85 percent, to an estimated 67.5 million in 1996, according to the American Association of Health Plans, the Washington, D.C.-based managed-care trade group (Lynch, 1998a). Meanwhile, continuing industry consolidation, increased competition in local markets, and the growing interest and participation of consumers in healthcare decision making are also helping redefine the landscape of healthcare delivery in the United States.

HISTORY OF MANAGING HEALTH

"For many years, we have bred a certain type of physician," observes Gordon K. Norman, M.D., vice president and medical plan director for PacifiCare in Cyprus, California (Lynch, 1998b). These physicians, he notes, were highly individualistic. They cherished their autonomy and resisted any infringement on it. They worked alone, preferring not to delegate or share responsibilities with others. Their relationship with their patients tended to be authoritarian; as physicians, they knew what was best. Under **fee-for-service** medicine, in which the payer paid a fee for each service, physicians had no reason to be concerned about the costs of care; rather, they had every incentive not to care. These traits, says Norman, are all part of a "very strong legacy from the professional guild tradition of medicine and the apprenticeship form of training" (Lynch, 1998b).

Following World War II, when the demand for healthcare was high and the supply was low, the cost of care began a dizzying ascent. The federal government provided free-flowing funds for the building of new healthcare facilities. Providers at this point had unlimited power: no competition and no financial risk in a fee-for-service market.

During the "Great Society" period of the 1960s, healthcare became available to all people, regardless of their ability to pay. **Medicare**, a federal program of assistance with healthcare costs for the over-65 elderly and some disabled persons, and **Medicaid**, a joint federal-state program designed to pay for indigents' healthcare, was established. However, even with a population insured by Medicare and Medicaid, providers still worked in a fee-for-service environment. They now had to shift costs, charging their insured patients more to cover the losses incurred from the nonpaying or underinsured patients. Medical costs continued to rise.

The passage in 1973 of the federal HMO Act gave **managed care** companies the ability to compete in the national healthcare market. The idea of grouping providers into exclusive networks and paying them less while guaranteeing them a larger number of patients slowly penetrated the healthcare industry. It also marked the beginning of competition, which was compounded by the 1983 diagnostically related groups (DRGs) legislation, outlining what the government would reimburse hospitals for Medicare patients (Kachnowski, 1997).

Medical costs continued to rise in the 1980s, leaving employers and other healthcare purchasers little choice but to add levels of management to medical care. These levels included utilization review, case management under fee-for-service care, and financial incentives for physicians under managed care. The mid-1980s saw the implementation of a new system of reimbursement, a **prospective payment system (PPS)**, for Medicare clients in hospitals. Under this system, the hospital received a flat rate based on DRGs for each patient admitted. This created an incentive to decrease the length of a hospital stay as a way of reducing costs. The expenditures still grew and began to influence the competitive edge of U.S. businesses because employers bore the burden of health insurance benefits for their employees (Huber, 1996).

By the early 1990s, the focus of the healthcare crisis had expanded to include access to care. Millions of Americans had no healthcare coverage. The first 5 years of the decade saw double-digit healthcare inflation. Between 1989 and 1990, healthcare costs rose 10.5 percent (U.S. Bureau of the Census, 1993). In 1991, healthcare spending rose by 11.4 percent to reach $751.8 billion, or 13.2 percent of the gross domestic product. The General Accounting Office's 1994 data projected that by the year 2000 about 17 percent of the gross domestic product would be spent on healthcare (Porter-O'Grady & Wilson, 1995, p. 8). Escalating costs and a growing uninsured population continued to strain individual, employer, and government budgets. The number of uninsured Americans was approximately 43 million in 1994 and continued to expand by more than 1 million per year (American Nurses Association, 1994).

Employers bearing the majority of healthcare costs began turning to managed-care organizations based on the assumption that managed-care plans lowered costs for payers while maintaining an acceptable level of services and quality of care. HMOs proliferated in the early 1990s because an employer could agree to pay no more than a fixed fee for a given group of employees and dependents. The HMO industry was now taking on the financial risk of a given population and was gaining control of the trillion-dollar healthcare business.

Although many persons bemoan managed care and its emphasis on cost containment and efficiency, they fail to recognize an important benefit that managed care can bring to the delivery of healthcare. Managed care is the one force big enough to help reshape the healthcare system so that it delivers better value to Americans. In 1995, a report produced by the Pew Health Professions Commission, "Critical Challenges: Revitalizing the Health Professions for the Twenty-First Century," recognized the enormous changes sweeping the healthcare system. According to the report, the new healthcare delivery system concentrates on delivering care that improves quality, lowers costs, and enhances patient satisfaction (Lynch, 1998a). Effective information management is a crucial component of any improvement activity. Delivering the right information to those most directly involved in decision making influences the outcomes of healthcare delivery.

In the environment of managing health, providers are expected to take responsibility for whole populations, not only to cure people of their ills but also to prevent illness when possible and to provide a continuum of care. Providers are expected to deliver high-quality care that responds to patients' needs and preferences and to be cognizant of the attendant costs. To practice effectively under these conditions, physicians and other healthcare professionals must develop new skills, competencies, and attitudes toward their work. In fact, they must reinvent their professional culture.

CULTURE CHANGE

Part of the dissatisfaction with managed care arises from uneasiness with the unknown and from the fact that all transitions are painful. Basing decisions on quality improvement and accountability is a significant cultural shift. Just as consumers have come to expect and even demand information about services and products purchased, they also have come to expect that the healthcare industry, including physicians and allied health professionals, will gather information and make it available to help people understand what high quality is and who the high-quality providers are. That is an uncomfortable change for most providers and patients. According to Mark Smith, president and CEO of the California HealthCare Foundation, it is uncomfortable for providers because it is the first time they have ever been held accountable (Lynch, 1998b). Most patients find it uncomfortable to walk into their surgeon's office feeling the same skepticism with which they would approach a car dealer.

The cultural shift is difficult for many to accept because it refutes the belief many hold that costs should not enter into the decision to provide healthcare to those in need. If a treatment or intervention has any chance of producing some benefit, no matter how small, then the practitioner's duty, as the patient's advocate, is to make sure that the patient gets the treatment. The goal for controlling costs is to develop information that can assist those charged with making such decisions. In the 1990s, and more so in the future, practitioners must pay close attention to every aspect of their practice, including the costs of resources used to produce and deliver interventions and the effects of these interventions on patients. As financial limits on resources increase, professionals need to be more informed about the likely consequences of their decisions.

Cost-effective delivery of care is not a new thought. In 1860, Florence Nightingale emphasized the cost-effective delivery of care and the use of data to prove this to the public:

> These statistics would show subscribers how their money was being spent, what amount of good was really being done with it, or whether the money was doing mischief rather than good. . . . [Statistics] would enable us to ascertain the mortality in different hospitals, as well as from different diseases and injuries among the classes which enter hospitals in different countries, and in different districts of the same country. They could enable us to ascertain how much of each year of life is wasted by illness.
>
> —Anderson, 1996, p. 29.

Much consumer distrust of managed care results from limited knowledge or understanding of the implications of the transition in the delivery of care. The media have not been helpful in communicating the positive aspects of managed care. A research study (Bernard & Shulkin,

1998) to determine the effect of the media on the public's perception of managed care reveals that in only 8 percent of cases did articles have a positive influence on readers. Two-thirds of the articles presented such unfavorable messages that readers were unlikely to join a managed-care organization. As with any cultural change, the shift in healthcare delivery has caused problems, but the positive aspects of quality care and the focus on wellness must be communicated to the public and providers.

Because managed care is still relatively new, debate about its merits will continue for some time. As long as data on clinical outcomes and other quality measures remain sparse, issues of quality in managed care will remain controversial. Unfortunately, the types of outcome studies needed to supply data are complex and take a long time to complete. In the meantime, the press will continue to provide the public with information about managed care. This information will inevitably play an important role in influencing people's decisions about their healthcare coverage.

DEFINITION OF MANAGED CARE

"Managed care" is a term used historically to define a new type of health financing system, namely, a capitated system as opposed to a fee-for-service system, and the controls introduced to manage the new set of risk relationships. **Capitation** is a payment plan that prepays a fixed amount of money per person to provide all the care needed for a specified population. The population might be, for example, all Medicaid patients in one state, all members of a union, or all employees in one manufacturing plant. If the designated population does not utilize the set amount, the provider gains financially. If the set amount is not adequate for the designated population, the provider loses financially. The provider of the care is at financial risk. In a fee-for-service traditional payment plan, the provider bills for each encounter or service rendered. The limitations determine the type, amount, or number of fees. The payer of the care is at financial risk. At the most general level, managed care refers to controls over medical costs introduced by managing costs, the utilization of services, and the employee/employer benefit package. The key word in managed care is "control."

Managed care is a system for providing healthcare that is managed by a physician designated by the patient as a **primary care provider (PCP)**. Managed-care systems offer a package of healthcare benefits, explicit standards for selection of healthcare providers, formal programs for ongoing quality assurance and utilization review, and significant incentives for their members to use providers and procedures associated with the plan.

The focus is on wellness, not illness. Goals for managed care include health maintenance, cost control for healthcare, and utilization of the least costly setting to provide healthcare. The PCP's role is to provide health maintenance exams and other routine health screenings to help maintain or improve the patient's health. When specialty care is essential, a referral is made to a specialist for any care beyond the realm of the PCP. The cost of care above and beyond the capitation fees collected is the financial responsibility of the PCP. The PCP is the gatekeeper in managed care. This system prevents fragmentation of care and duplication of services. Managed-care advocates view this approach to the delivery of care as a more holistic approach, as the patient is treated as a person, not a disease process.

TYPES OF MANAGED-CARE PLANS

According to the American Nurses Association (1994), three basic types of managed care organizations exist: health maintenance organizations (HMOs), **preferred provider organizations (PPOs)**, and **point-of-service plans (POSs)**.

A federally funded HMO has three characteristics: an organized system for providing health care in a geographic area; an agreed-on set of basic and supplemental health maintenance and treatment services; and a voluntarily enrolled group of people.

A PPO contracts with independent providers for negotiated, discounted fees for services provided to members. Usually, the contract provides significantly better benefits for services received from preferred providers, thus encouraging covered persons to use these providers. Covered persons are allowed benefits for nonparticipating providers' services, but with significant copayments.

A POS provides a set of healthcare benefits and offers a range of health services; however, the members have the choice of using either the managed-care program or out-of-program services each time they seek care. Members incur substantially higher costs if they select a provider outside the network.

ADVANTAGES AND DISADVANTAGES OF MANAGED CARE

In theory, managed care is a cost-effective method of delivering quality healthcare. Patients receive care through a single seamless system as they move from wellness to illness and back to wellness again. Continuity of care, prevention, and early intervention are stressed. The management of the health needs of individuals controls the cost of healthcare.

In reality, however, in many managed-care environments, managed care is seen not as a system of organizing patient care, but as a mechanism of financing healthcare. Some providers are adopting cost-cutting tools developed by managed-care organizations, such as early hospital discharge without thorough follow-up. "Drive-through delivery" is an ex-

TABLE 10.1 ▶ ADVANTAGES AND DISADVANTAGES OF MANAGED CARE

Advantages	Disadvantages
Focus is on providing higher-quality care through more efficient, cost-effective means.	Patients' choices are often financially restricted to using the managed-care system's providers and other services.
Preventive measures such as well-baby checks emphasize wellness.	Certain procedures are either not covered or have limited reimbursement compared to traditional insurance plans.
Capping provider payments and curtailing overutilization of the health system control healthcare costs.	Clinical care decisions can be affected by the provisions of the managed-care system.
Discounted insurance rates decrease healthcare costs.	
Seamless continuity of care can be provided through a single gatekeeper physician.	

ample of this practice. Providers encouraged by managed-care incentives were sending mothers and newborns home within 12 to 24 hours of normal delivery. Payors were stressing cost reduction without adequate regard to appropriate follow-up care, complete assessment of the health of the mother and baby, and adequate teaching to ensure that the mother had learned needed skills for caring for her new baby. The public outcry over arbitrarily set limits for hospitalization for mothers and infants prompted state and federal legislators to recognize that mothers and newborns require careful assessment of their needs for care and appropriate home care following delivery. An arbitrary time limit cannot be set for all patients. A summary of the advantages and disadvantages of managed care appears in *Table 10.1*.

NEED FOR QUALITY DATA

Managed care is not possible without the use of advanced information management technology because the practice of managed care depends on a wealth of detailed information that can come only from automated systems (Simpson, 1997). Information about membership enrollment, plan benefits, diagnostic and intervention codes, providers, and reimbursement arrangements must be gathered and processed. Gathering quality data is vital for producing quality outcomes. If data are incorrect, incomplete, and late, providers make uninformed or incorrect decisions about patient care. Information systems are extremely useful because of their ability to rearrange or summarize data for subsequent analysis; however, they cannot turn bad data into truth, hence, the saying, "Garbage in, garbage out." Data retrieved from a database are only as good as the data entered into the database.

At a famous hospital in the Northeast, the CEO and vice-presidents examined their referral patterns of obstetrical/gynecological physicians to the hospital. They wanted to know where their patients came from so that they could concentrate the hospital's marketing efforts appropriately. When they generated the reports, they found to their astonishment that fully 50 percent of their patients were referred from a single ZIP code. Even more amazing, that ZIP code contained only three physicians, two of whom were about to retire. They then talked to the employees in the obstetrical department who entered the data. One person said, "You know, many patients are close to delivery or in emergent condition when they hit the door here. I have to get them registered immediately before we can order any medications, labs, etc. So, when I can't get their ZIP code, a required field for registration, I enter my own ZIP code to fill in the field" (Stahlhut, 1996, p. 2). From a data entry perspective this behavior makes perfect sense and happens often, but from a management perspective it leads to poor decisions.

CODING DATA

To gather quality information, data are codified to enhance and simplify the categorizing of health and disease. The process of using data to generate codes is complex and somewhat subjective. Data in a health record, for example, require interpretation before a diagnostic code is assigned. The act of interpretation affects the codes selected. To ensure that the process results in the codes best suited to the task at hand, those who understand that task should be involved in the code selection process. This involvement does not always occur because professionals are often removed from the coding process. According to Coiera (1997), the quality of coding improves:

- The closer it occurs to the point of information capture
- If the individuals involved in the coding understand how the coded data are to be used
- If the staff members doing the coding benefit from the coding

Comprehension of and involvement in the coding process by allied health professionals improve the quality of the information used for reimbursement, management decision making, and research. The most common healthcare coding systems used in the United States are diagnostically related groups (DRGs), Current Procedural Terminology (CPT), the International Classification of Disease (ICD-9), and the Systematized Nomenclature of Medicine (SNOMED).

In the mid-1980s the government made an attempt to curb the rising cost of healthcare through a system of prospective, rather than retrospective, healthcare payment for all Medicare recipients. Other insurance or third-party payors soon followed suit. This system of prospective payment finds its base in **diagnostically related groups (DRGs)**. Based on the DRG code, a provider (physician or hospital) receives reimbursement at a set amount for a specific condition, stipulated ahead of time.

Each DRG takes the principal diagnosis or procedure responsible for a patient's admission and gives a corresponding cost weight. This weight is applied according to a formula to determine the amount that should be paid to an institution for a patient with a particular DRG. Hospitals responded to these restrictions by instituting cost-cutting measures and by drastically reducing hospital stays.

Current Procedural Terminology (CPT) is a coding of procedures and services performed by physicians. The purpose of the terminology is to describe medical, surgical, and diagnostic services in a reliable and consistent manner. CPT is also useful for administrative management purposes such as claims processing and for the development of guidelines for medical care review. The uniform language is applicable to medical education and research by providing a useful basis for local, regional, and national utilization comparisons.

The ninth edition of the **International Classification of Disease (ICD)** classifies morbidity and mortality information from nations throughout the world for statistical purposes, indexing of hospital records by disease and operations, data storage, and data retrieval. Although not originally intended for hospital use, ICD coding systems have been modified throughout several editions to reflect the level of detail necessary for hospitals. Physicians have been required by law to submit diagnosis codes for Medicare reimbursement since the passage of the Medicare Catastrophic Coverage Act of 1988 (St. Anthony's, 1995, viii). This act requires physician offices to include the appropriate diagnosis codes when billing for services provided to Medicare beneficiaries on or after April 1, 1989. The Health Care Financing Administration designated ICD-9-CM as the coding system physicians must use. Most other major classification systems endeavor to make their systems compatible with ICD so that data coded in these systems can be mapped directly to ICD codes.

In 1993 the World Health Organization published the tenth edition of this classification system, ICD-10. This version contains the greatest number of changes in the history of ICD. It expands the list for specialty-based adaptations and contains lists that cover topics beyond morbidity and mortality. For example, there are classifications of medical and surgical procedures and disablement. ICD-10 was adopted for use in Europe in the 1990s, and implementation in the United States is expected in the year 2000.

The Systematized Nomenclature of Medicine (SNOMED) is intended as a general-purpose, comprehensive, and computer-processable terminology to represent and index all of the events found in the medical record. SNOMED allows the composition of complex terms from simpler terms and incorporates virtually all of the ICD-9-CM terms and codes.

Computerized coding saves time and results in higher-quality codes. According to a 1996 study (Hohnloser et al., 1996), computer-assisted use of ICD-9 codes improved the completeness of the codes by 55 percent. The increase of accuracy rose from 41 to 92 percent, and computerization reduced coding time by 50 percent.

INVISIBILITY OF ALLIED HEALTH PROFESSIONS IN DATA COLLECTION

ICD, DRG, CPT, and SNOMED codification systems are all medically based and do not reflect the practice, interventions, and outcomes attributable to allied health professions. Using information from the coding data sets is helpful in making purchase decisions, allocating resources, making comparisons in a search for best practices, and making policy decisions. It has been said that information is power. If allied health professionals are to influence the delivery of healthcare in managed-care environments, an information infrastructure similar to those used by the power structures that design and control the delivery and purchasing of healthcare in the United States must be developed.

In his first annual report, William Farr (1807–1883), the first medical statistician for the General Register Office of England and Wales, noted:

> The advantages of a uniform statistical nomenclature, however imperfect, are so obvious, that it is surprising that no attention has been paid to its enforcement in Bills of Mortality. Each disease has, in many instances, been denoted by three or four terms, and each term has been applied to as many different diseases: vague, inconvenient names have been employed or complications have been registered instead of primary diseases. The nomenclature is of as much importance in this department of enquiry as weights and measures in the physical sciences, and should be settled without delay.
>
> —ICD-10, 1993.

Standardizing language both within and across professions is necessary for documenting the value of allied health professions to the delivery of healthcare.

MEASURING MANAGED CARE

The quality of healthcare is always difficult to measure. Various accrediting bodies attempt to quantify quality in the organizations they accredit. The **National Committee on Quality Assurance (NCQA)** accredits qualified managed-care organizations. NCQA accreditation employs both on- and offsite audits. The onsite records audit utilizes CPT and ICD-9 codes and the **Health Plan Employer Data and Information Set (HEDIS)**. HEDIS is a set of standardized performance measures designed to ensure that purchasers and consumers have the information they need to compare the performance of managed healthcare plans reli-

> BOX 10.1   HEDIS PERFORMANCE MEASURES
>
> • Cancer screening
> • Checkups after delivery
> • Eye exams for diabetics
> • Follow-up after mental illness
> • Prenatal care
> • Childhood immunizations
> • Educating smokers
> • Flu shots for the elderly

ably. The performance measures in HEDIS are related to many significant public health issues such as cancer, heart disease, smoking, asthma, mental health, and diabetes *(Box 10.1)*. HEDIS also employs a member satisfaction survey. Managed-care organizations, coalitions of managed-care organizations, and healthcare purchasers use HEDIS measures to evaluate the quality of health plans. The 1999 database reflects the performance of 490 companies, 331 of which are HMOs and 159 POSs. Although the availability of information is welcome, significant problems still remain in trying to collate and compare the data across such reports.

TRACKING OUTCOMES INFORMATION

To be evaluated in managing healthcare, quality must be stated in measurable terms. An outcome is the end result of a course of treatment; for example, the patient can walk normally again. Outcomes systems track the treatment plan and resource utilization to determine whether something could be changed in the future to improve the outcome so that, for example, the patient can walk normally again within 3 weeks instead of 10. The ability to state outcomes in measurable terms facilitates quality care and intelligent allocation of resources.

It is the ability to measure the resources used over the course of a physician's treatment plan that will set apart one hospital system from the rest. By delivering healthcare efficiently and improving patient outcomes, the best hospitals also will be the most financially successful. Eventually, hospital management will price services based on the clinical risk of a population, such as knowing how much it will cost to care for 400 employees in a manufacturing plant.

WELLNESS INFORMATION DECREASES COSTS

Managed care emphasizes wellness education and is economically driven by capitation to provide patients with easy access to information on a wide variety of issues, including preventive care, disease management information, weight management, and smoking cessation programs. Whereas traditional thinking meant treating sickness, avoiding risk, giving episodic and emergency care, and using provider-based services payment, the new thinking means promoting wellness, managing risk, providing comprehensive and preventive care, and finally, using managed care and managed costs. To help address these concerns, hospital networks are being linked to provide full access to information services. For example, interactive voice access to medical hotlines in the native language of the patient; nurse triage services, which have been proven to lower the costs of healthcare; and wellness information services available through both managed-care organizations' and employers' Internet and intranet low-cost access are now underway.

Good health is strongly dependent on lifestyle choices made by the patient. Some employers institute tough standards to ensure that their employees make healthier lifestyle choices. This practice is controversial, but the bottom line is at stake. In some cases, injuries incurred while playing high-risk sports or practicing other high-risk behaviors, such as not wearing a seat belt, are not covered. Other employers, while permitting high-risk behavior, use higher deductibles instead. The patient must have health, wellness, and risk information in order to make the correct choices.

In educating employees about their healthcare choices and lifestyles, many managed-care companies now employ a 24-hour, toll-free health information access line or e-mail system staffed by a registered nurse. Nurses can address medical problems and refer patients to programs for smoking cessation, alcoholism rehabilitation, or weight management. Other helplines are more sophisticated. In Colorado, the QualMed plan utilizes high-tech nurses with access to the HMO's database. They consult electronic patient records over the phone and apply clinical pathways in lieu of a physician consultation.

At the Oxford Health Plan in Connecticut, queries addressed to the patient database identify asthma patients, and pertinent health information along with oxygen flow monitoring meters are mailed to these patients. The plan claims that hospitalization of Medicaid asthma patients has fallen by a third (Edwards & Sandberg, 1997). Companies and payers encourage these preliminary steps as a way to provide information to those who would otherwise go to the emergency room or schedule unneeded treatments with their primary care physicians. In Oregon, Access Health services helped Medicaid patients cut emergency room visits by half. By using their health services, they also prevent an average of one physician visit a year, providing a savings of $184 per patient. Kaiser Permanente in Silicon Valley, California, provides online appointment scheduling by patients. Using a personal identification number (PIN) to access a Web site, members can also search 30,000 pages of disease-specific information; participate in discussion groups; send questions to a nurse, pharmacist, or specialist; or order prescription refills or over-the-counter medication from an online drugstore (Schneider, 1997). The Comprehensive Health Enhancement Support System (CHESS) is a network of home health workstations created by the University of Wisconsin. This network for people with AIDS, breast cancer, and other problems provides links to other patients, care providers, medical information libraries, and other resources (Essex, 1999).

CASE MANAGEMENT

Patients with chronic diseases, who are the major healthcare consumers, have the most to gain from preventive care and ongoing counseling and management. Asthma sufferers whose routine treatment used to be delivered in emergency rooms are now avoiding crises through concerted education and preventive care, at significant savings to their insurers. The same is true of those with diabetes and hypertension. The diseases themselves are much less costly to manage than the crises they provoke.

"Case management" and "disease management" are terms describing a process of continuously analyzing, evaluating, and improving the value of healthcare delivery across the spectrum of care settings for individuals and identified populations. **Case management** most often refers to individuals requiring intensive, usually noninstitutional care for a particular illness, condition, or injury over a period of time to optimize the quality of life and allow the patient to achieve normal or partial functioning. **Disease management** is a proactive, integrated care approach that includes identification and stratification of patients or populations of patients at risk, such as those who have chronic diseases or are likely to suffer a catastrophic event, as well as implementation of preventive programs and treatments to prevent or minimize crises. Supported by sophisticated analytical software, healthcare executives can analyze large numbers of patients for current and future risk factors to allocate precious healthcare dollars more efficiently.

Both case management and disease management utilize the same data to make decisions concerning quality of care and outcomes measures. Increasingly, clinical disease and case management products enable clinicians to standardize and manage patient care throughout large, integrated delivery systems. Although improvements in the quality of patient care might be justification enough to warrant investment, case management strategies are also saving money.

Some managed-care insurers focus on population or community-based healthcare management. These companies aim to coordinate care throughout all health delivery entities to improve both clinical and financial outcomes. They enrich their database information by incorporating personal health profiles. They emphasize the importance of factoring in such information as personal and family medical histories, health habits, environment, and culture, as these strongly influence the development of chronic disease or a catastrophic event such as diabetes or a heart attack. Managed-care products are focusing more on prediction and prevention based on the theory that predicting which persons are most likely to develop a particular disease or suffer a catastrophic event provides an opportunity to do something about it.

Information provided by feeder systems such as admission/discharge/transfer, order entry/results reporting, patient accounting, and laboratory, pharmacy, and radiology departments is required for appropriate, accurate, and up-to-date clinical and financial patient information. These systems are an integral part of case management, as they provide the foundation for concurrent evaluation of care.

Critical paths and clinical protocols, used as methods of clinical practice management, move beyond traditional care plans to integrate with multidisciplinary clinical documentation. Critical paths are an abridged version of a diagnosis-specific, multidisciplinary plan of care. These paths incorporate critical events and interventions that must occur in a given time frame and sequence to achieve specific patient outcomes. Clinical protocols are guidelines for medical interventions for specific clinical conditions based on approved standards of care. These guidelines may be time oriented or sequential, but usually they do not incorporate overall patient outcomes (Remmlinger et al., 1995). To realize the full benefits of critical paths and clinical protocols, they must be automated. Integration with feeder systems is required to enable interactive alerts for duplicated or nonstandard procedures, drug interactions, abnormal findings, or delayed or poor patient outcomes. Concurrent alerts to variances from the prescribed treatment plan or expected outcome can trigger quality management issues for follow-up, as well as changes in the treatment plan without delaying care.

Outcome analysis capabilities are required for case managers to understand variances. Outcome tracking is required for review of critical paths and clinical protocols, evaluation of provider performance, and review of clinical outcomes in the context of utilization of clinical and financial resources. Information technology is critical in implementing a comprehensive and effective case management process.

ROLE OF PROVIDERS IN MANAGING HEALTH INFORMATION

Managed care provides the impetus for each healthcare discipline to prove its worth. The best method for achieving this is through the proactive use of information technology. To capture information that measures the effect of interventions on outcomes, codifying contributions in a standardized language, using agreed-on definitions, and entering data are all essential.

Deciding what data to collect is an important issue. Practicing without good data is no longer a valid option. Start with quality indicators reported through HEDIS and benchmark against other facilities in the region. When suboptimal quality occurs, thoughtful interdisciplinary examination of the processes involved can be undertaken to improve methods.

Information systems can support the goals of patient education with printouts of instructions and systems with flags and alarms that remind case managers to follow up with specific patients or patient populations. In addition, information technology enables care managers to interact with clients over interactive TV and the Internet to provide teaching, monitoring, and follow-up care.

Within the parameters of each healthcare discipline, professionals can:

- Assess the patient to determine health status and risks, unhealthy lifestyles, minor health problems, and health education needs of patients and their families
- Provide support and reassurance while caring for present or potential health problems
- Advocate for primary and preventive care services

Managed-care organizations that value quality and recognize the importance of prevention, wellness, and early intervention can benefit from expertise in a variety of roles. In turn, providers can help guide managed-care companies to focus on providing a full range of quality, cost-effective services.

SUMMARY

According to Edward O'Neil, executive director of the Pew Health Professions Commission, "this is a period of great dislocation and enormous opportunity in health care in the United States. What strikes many as a chaotic, confusing, and conflicting change from the past is, in fact, a process of fundamental realignment of purposes, processes, and people" (O'Neil, 1999, p. 10). The healthcare delivery system is undergoing a dramatic change, shifting from uncontrolled and unmonitored care to managed care.

In the past, healthcare was a collection of small private practices and solo community-based institutions that, for the most part, controlled their own destinies. They were exempt from public or private control beyond the self-regulation of the professions themselves. This autonomy created a burgeoning financial burden on the payors for healthcare. In an effort to decrease costs while increasing quality, the marketplace has redirected the management of healthcare delivery, principally through managed-care organizations. Market values for healthcare revolve around issues of cost, consumer satisfaction, and quality. The focus of care is also moving from individual recipients of care to a broader social context of improving the health of overall populations through effective public health interventions and quality health outcomes.

Information technology has the potential to arrange healthcare resources to best serve the patient and create a knowledge-based system that can continually improve the quality of outcomes. Gathering significant, quality data will produce meaningful outcome measurements to assist with the decisions concerning the interventions most effective in improving outcomes. Allied healthcare providers need to own the process of change by managing outcomes and costs, creating the best workforce mix to produce desired outcomes.

▶ LEARNING EXERCISES

1. Discussion questions
   - Historically, who determined the cost of healthcare?
   - Who pays for the majority of healthcare?
   - How have rising costs created a cultural shift in healthcare delivery?
   - Is cost an issue when determining the quality of care?
   - What part do the media play in making healthcare choices?
   - Does each allied health profession need to develop a specialized language to prove its worth in managed care?
   - What part does evidence-based healthcare play in managed care?
   - What is the difference between fee-for-service and capitation payment plans?
2. Debate the advantages and disadvantages of managed care.
3. Interview a physician concerning the impact of managed-care data on his or her practice.
4. Interview allied health providers concerning their role in determining indicators for quality care.
5. Use the Internet to find HEDIS information. Is the information complete and understandable enough for consumers and employers to make informed decisions about healthcare providers?

References

American Nurses Association. (1994). *Managed care: Challenges and opportunities for nursing* [brochure]. Washington, DC: Author.
Anderson, R. (1996). One nursing minimum data set: A key to nursing's future. In M. E. Mills, C. A. Romano, & B. R. Heller (pp. 28–31). *Information management in nursing and health care*. Springhouse, PA: Springhouse.

Bernard, D. B., & Shulkin, D. J. (1998). The media vs. managed health care: Are we seeing a full court press? *Archives of Internal Medicine, 158*, 2109–2111.

Coiera, E. (1997). *Guide to medical informatics, the Internet and telemedicine.* London: Chapman & Hall.

Edwards, G., & Sandberg, L. (1997). The role of information technology in the evolution of health care delivery. *Proceedings of Healthcare Information and Management Systems Society, 2,* 11–21.

Essex, D. (1999, February). Life line: Consumer informatics has gone beyond patient education on the Web. *Healthcare Informatics,* 119–121.

Hohnloser, J. H., Kadlec, P., & Puerner, F. (1996). Coding clinical information: Analysis of clinicians using computerized coding. *Methods of Information in Medicine, 35*(2), 104–107.

Huber, D. (1996). *Leadership and nursing care management.* Philadelphia: W. B. Saunders.

ICD-10 (1993). *International statistical classification of diseases and related health problems* (10th rev.). Geneva: World Health Organization.

Kachnowski, S. (1997, January). A system long overdue. *Healthcare Informatics,* 27–33.

Lynch, E. (1998a, Summer). Growth of managed care. *Front & Center, 2*(4), 1–8.

Lynch, E. (1998b, Summer). Interview with Mark D. Smith, MD, MBA. *Front & Center, 2*(4), 4.

Marietti, C. (1999, March). Seize the disease! *Healthcare Informatics,* 43–54.

O'Neil, E. (1999, January/February). The opportunity that is nursing. *Nursing and Health Care Perspectives, 20*(1), 10–14.

Porter-O'Grady, T., & Wilson, C. K. (1995). *The leadership revolution in health care: Altering systems, changing behaviors.* Gaithersburg, MD: Aspen.

Remmlinger, E., Ault, S., & Hanrahan, L. (1995, Winter). Information technology implications of case management. *The Journal of the Healthcare Information and Management Systems Society, 9*(1), 21–28.

Schneider, P. (1997, August). Patient Informatics is growing. *Healthcare Informatics,* 26.

Schneider, P. (1998, April). Kaiser Permanente seeks salvation in IT. *Healthcare Informatics,* 72–78.

Simpson, R. L. (1997). Take advantage of managed care opportunities. *Nursing Management, 28*(3), 24–25.

St. Anthony's ICD-9-CM code book for physician payment. (1995). Reston, VA: St. Anthony.

Stahlhut, R. (1996, Spring). Avoiding the garbage-in→garbage-out phenomenon. *AMSA Task Force Quarterly,*

U.S. Bureau of the Census. (1993). *Statistical abstract of the United States* (113th ed.). Washington, DC: U.S. Government Printing Office.

11

Electronic Communications

JAMES LEJA AND KATHLEEN M. YOUNG

Key Words continued on page 186

Packet switching
Personal digital assistant
  (PDA)
Plug-in programs
Search engine
Subject directory
Synchronous communication

Transmission Control Protocol/
  Interworking Protocol (TCP/IP)
Uniform resource locator (URL)
USENET
Voice recognition
Web site evaluation
World Wide Web (Web)

LEARNING OBJECTIVES

By the end of this chapter, you will be able to:
▶ Describe the basics of connecting to the Internet
▶ Describe the development of computers
▶ Describe the common tools and applications associated with
  electronic communications
▶ Describe issues and solutions related to the security and
  confidentiality of electronic data
▶ Evaluate Web sites
▶ Utilize the Web for professional purposes
▶ Apply various communication technologies to health and human
  services activities

A state public health official uses her automated statistical program to interface with the World Wide Web (Web) in order to compare the most recent data on deaths due to sudden infant death syndrome (SIDS) in her state with data that have been added systematically to the state database during the previous year. During that period, the public health department initiated a special campaign to educate hospital officials, health professionals, and new parents on the importance of the infant sleeping position in reducing SIDS. Working through the Internet, a task force representing health professional groups, managed-care plans, hospitals, public libraries, and community service organizations developed and implemented a comprehensive statewide plan. Rather than meeting in a common geographic location, the task force members communicated through e-mail and teleconferencing. Web-based multimedia bulletins were developed summarizing the results of research implicating the sleep position in SIDS and illustrating correct and incorrect sleeping positions. On the Web, the task force published long-distance learning programs focusing on sleep positions and produced inexpensive CD-ROMs for parents taking infants home from the hospital. The task force also encouraged hospitals and clinics to provide workstations and kiosks so that parents coming in for well childcare visits could view the information and access other Web sites on newborn care. CD-ROMs were given to public libraries, clinics, and hospitals to encourage participation and provide access to as many people as possible.

Linking the SIDS data to other statewide information resources through the Web, the state public health official explores several possible explanations for the lack of reduction in in-home SIDS in certain jurisdictions. She explores language barriers (the SIDS educational material was produced in English and Spanish only) and less frequent visits to the clinicians who provided reminders. Because the incidence of SIDS is higher in jurisdictions with a lower percentage of immunized babies, this latter explanation seems plausible. The official notifies the task force members of her findings through e-mail. At a teleconference, the task force decides to add additional members from the identified communities to target interventions in these areas.

This scenario captures some of the potential use of electronic communications in the healthcare environment. The professionals in the scenario communicated through e-mail and teleconferencing, researched through automated statistical packages and the Web, and developed Web-based multimedia bulletins and CD-ROM programs. Many other applications also exist to communicate relevant information to human service professionals and the public. This chapter focuses on the use of computer and other electronic technologies in the delivery of health and human services.

A BIT OF HISTORY

According to the Jones Telecommunications and Multimedia Encyclopedia (1999), computing actually has quite a long history. In 3000 BC, the abacus was invented in Asia Minor to assist merchants with trading transactions. In 1642, 18-year-old Blaise Pascal invented the first numerical calculating machine in Paris to help his tax collector father with his duties. Charles Babbage designed the analytical engine, the first computer. He was frustrated with the many errors he found while examining calculations for the Royal Astronomical Society and in 1833, with the assistance of Augusta Ada King, the first female programmer, he developed a steam-powered machine that followed instructions on punched cards. In the last years of the 1800s, Herman Hollerith improved on the punched card concept and reduced the amount of time necessary to compute the U.S. Census from 10 years to 6 weeks. With his invention, he began the Computing-Tabulating-Recording Company, which later became International Business Machines (IBM).

With the onset of the Second World War, the Germans, British, and Americans all sought to develop computers to exploit their country's potential strategic importance. In 1945, spurred by the war effort, a team of electrical engineers at the Moore School of Electrical Engineering of the University of Pennsylvania in Philadelphia, completed a secret project for the U.S. Army, developing a calculator called ENIAC (Electronic Numerator, Integrator, Analyzer, and Computer). ENIAC incorporated 17,468 vacuum tubes, weighed 30 tons, covered about 1000 square feet of flooring, and consumed 130–140 kilowatts of electricity. It could do 5000 addition and 360 multiplication problems per second.

In these early days of computers, when it was necessary to access information (data), put information in (input), or send it out or print it (output), one had to enter the "computer room," an air-conditioned room with a wall-sized computer (the mainframe) and a large line printer. As time passed, these computer users, most often researchers, came up with ways to manipulate their data without actually being in the mainframe room (Dern, 1994). This required the development of remote terminals (monitors and keyboards) and printers connected to the main computer. Networks facilitated the interconnectivity. Networks, connected by lines, enabled data to flow back and forth from the main computer to the terminal, to the printer, or to another computer.

The first lines were wire cables that connected the computer, terminal, and printer. However, as the distance between terminals and computers grew, data flow gradually degraded. When these lines were strung from the terminal in one room down the hall to the computer room, the signal sometimes became so faint as it reached the computer that the computer couldn't "hear" the data input down the hall.

To gain greater distance with data flow, telephone lines replaced the cables. To connect the computer or terminal to another one much farther away, a **modem** (*mo*dulated-*dem*odulated) attached to the telephone line converted the signal into something usable by the computers communicating with one another.

This system worked well when one computer tried to communicate with another, but when thousands of computers tried to communicate with one another, congestion resulted. To solve this problem, researchers developed a method by which computers could take turns sharing the lines. This required the use of a **multiplexor**, a device situated between the telephone line and a group of computers that divides the line into fragments of a second, giving each user a small portion of time in turn (Dern, 1994).

In the late 1960s, a new approach to time-sharing was developed called **packet switching**. Essentially, the data stream was divided into small packets of information that were reassembled at the endpoint. Each packet of data contained the address or identification (ID) number of the computer to which it was sent. Because each packet had its own address, many lines could connect with a packet switch or node at each connection to form a network. The node, therefore, was the place where lines intersected to transfer data to other lines.

In the 1960s, the U.S. Defense Department created the Advanced Research Projects Agency (ARPA) in response to the cold war. "It was designed for purposes of military communication in a United States devastated by a Soviet nuclear strike. Originally, the Internet was a post-apocalypse command grid" (Tappendorf, 1995, p. 1). ARPA's responsibility was to maintain lines of communication in the event of a nuclear strike to enable scientists across the globe to communicate with one another. Consequently, **ARPAnet** was created, becoming the precursor to the Internet, the World Wide Web, and e-mail. Because the nodes in ARPAnet were computers, engineers could program them to do many tasks, including calculating the best route through the network. Another task engineered into the computer was the detection of places where packets were not reaching their intended target computer due to line breakage or packet switch crashing. The packet switches determined where the problem occurred and recalculated alternative routes to the target computer (Dern, 1994). ARPAnet initially used a **communications protocol** or set of rules, known as the "network control protocol (NCP)" to allow computers to communicate with one another with limited errors. As other networks developed, a heterogeneous method was needed to foster communication between different networks. The Defense Advanced Research Projects Agency (DARPA), recognizing this need, sponsored the development of a new protocol dubbed the **Transmission Control Protocol/Interworking Protocol (TCP/IP)**. TCP/IP enabled communication for projects that involved computers on different networks, packet radio, and ARPAnet. This entire transaction is now called the "Internet."

Dern (1994) points out that the **Internet** is such a worldwide entity that it cannot be simply defined. It includes over 2 million computers connected to networks at thousands of locations belonging to governments, educational institutions, businesses, organizations, and homes in over 100 countries where text, graphics, and audio information travel back and forth within seconds.

History of the World Wide Web

A further innovation made movement from one document to another on the Internet very simple. In 1989, at the European Particle Physics Laboratory (CERN), work was being done to create files that would link with other files (Coiera, 1997). CERN's innovation, **hypertext**, permits users to "click" on a **hyperlink** within a document and move to another document at a remote location. Multimedia capability added still and moving images and voice to the basic text of the Internet. This expanding global collection of interconnected information sources is known as the World Wide Web (Web). The advent of the user-friendly protocols of the Web triggered public interest in using the Internet. "It was probably a combination of improved ease of use, along with the amount of information available on the Web reaching a critical mass, that brought the Internet to the public's attention" (Coiera, 1997, p. 248).

HARDWARE AND SOFTWARE FOR CONNECTING

Although not designed to create expertise in computer hardware and software, this chapter presents basic concepts and ideas related to computers and communications. An understanding of basic terminology is necessary to understand the concepts. The computer, like the telephone, is a tool for communications. An in-depth understanding of computers is not necessary to know how to use them effectively to affect healthcare practice.

Connecting to the Internet

To understand the following information most easily, a connection to the Internet is helpful. The appropriate equipment, a connection, and an Internet account are required. Equipment can range from the sophisticated to the basic. If the user is affiliated with an organization, university, hospital, or other such entity, the equipment to communicate via the computer is probably already supplied. If not, the purchase of some equipment is helpful. Purchasing the right equipment requires some research. Any number of computer stores and magazines willingly offer advice. Many magazines provide advice on such topics as selecting the right processor, deciding how much random access memory (RAM) is needed, how large a hard drive is needed for information storage, the type of display or monitor desired, and the advisability of a CD-ROM, modem, or other devices. Colleagues who work with the technology daily are often willing to offer both their opinions and assistance.

One method of connecting to the Internet is by remote access. Communication from the home computer to the host Internet computer requires the use of a modem and a telephone line. The other type of connection is direct access, which directly links the local computer to the host computer.

The modem enables a computer to transmit information over a standard telephone line. The baud rate is the transmitting speed of data. The higher the baud rate, the faster the data transmission. Most modems today operate at 28.8 kilobits per second (K bps), 33.6 K bps, or 56 K bps. Faster modems are generally better because they reduce the amount of connection time. However, the modems at both ends of the communication must have the same speed to operate at maximum potential. Therefore, if one modem operates at 56 K bps but the other modem at only 33.6 K bps, the transmission can connect no faster than 33.6 K bps. In addition, static and interference on telephone lines can reduce transmission speed. Modems are either internal or external to the computer. An internal modem hides all wires. External modems are small boxes requiring external cables. New computer systems most often come with internal modems.

Without the appropriate software, modems will not work. Subscribers to an **Internet service provider (ISP)** are often provided with the appropriate connecting software. Companies such as America Online, Compuserv, and MCI Mail provide connecting software. Universities generally provide a floppy or CD-ROM disk to install all the needed software that automatically establishes the settings for students and faculty.

To use the Internet, an account is needed. Again, ISP services such as America Online provide an account for a fee. Once an Internet provider is selected, software selected, and the connection made, it is necessary to establish a username, user ID or a screen name, and a password to gain access to the Internet. In some communities, libraries or other public consortia have organized limited free remote access to the Internet for community members. The ISP provides directions for each of these steps or directions come with essential software.

When the user has "logged on" or connected to the Internet using a modem through a home telephone line, telephone calls cannot be sent or received. Heavy users of the Internet might choose to install a second line dedicated to the computer. While typical residential telephone lines work well, an integrated services digital network (ISDN) line may be available. Because this line is digital rather than analog, the speed of communication is much faster. However, because ISDN is not yet the standard, it is unavailable in many areas and tends to be more expensive. It also requires additional hardware.

For users directly connected to the Internet through their work organization, the organization usually establishes the account and assigns a username and password. With this configuration, the computer or terminal may be connected directly to the Internet through a **local area network (LAN)**, a group of computers and other devices scattered over a relatively small area and connected by a communications link that allows any device to interact with any other on the network (Microsoft Press, 1991). Instead of a modem, a network interface or Ethernet Card, developed by Xerox in 1976, links microcomputers. Additionally, libraries may have public access to the Internet. If a home and office computer is used, a difference in the data receiving speed may appear. A home machine is usually much slower.

METHODS OF ACCESSING INFORMATION

Common methods of accessing information on the Internet are electronic mail (e-mail), the file transfer protocol (FTP), USENET, listservs, chat rooms, and the World Wide Web. E-mail, USENET, and listservs are all types of **asynchronous communication**, in which there is a delay between sending and receiving (Carlton & Miller, 1999). For example, an e-mail message sent at 9 AM may not be looked at by the receiver until 5 PM that day. The receiver controls the time for viewing the message. This is particularly convenient for global communication among very different time zones. A chat room is an example of **synchronous communication** requiring a response at the time the message is sent, which may not always be convenient for the receiver.

E-Mail

E-mail (electronic mail) sends messages between computers across a network. The use of e-mail for communication is so widespread that using it is no longer an option but rather a professional responsibility. It is a useful tool because of its speed of transfer and almost universal accessibility. Most people now have access to an e-mail account and can send messages to other people's accounts regardless of what system they are using. The e-mail program creates messages, sending them to a corresponding server program. Programs such as Netscape's Messenger, Eudora, and Microsoft's Outlook Express, among many others, are popular e-mail programs. The more sophisticated ones maintain address books and files and allow users to send and receive messages in Hyper-Text Markup Language. Attaching files from word-processing programs such as Microsoft Word or WordPerfect to an e-mail message sends them to the e-mail recipient. E-mail addresses follow this convention: username@place.suffix (such as jleja@wmich.edu). More periods can separate the username (for example, james.leja), or place (for example, oncolink.upenn). Common suffixes are gov (government), com (commercial), edu (education), mil (military), and org (organization).

Mandl et al. (1998) state that e-mail between physicians and patients is proliferating. They suggest, for example, that a patient can use e-mail to make an appointment, or request information such as a list of low-fat foods, or specific information about insulin dosages. The physician can initiate an e-mail contact to convey educational information, for example, about SIDS.

Security and confidentiality of e-mail is a concern. When dealing with sensitive data, such as medical information or other confidential information, others may intercept the message. One way of ensuring that e-mail messages are secure is to use encryption or authentication software. According to Mandl and colleagues (1998), the most current, best-developed technology for encrypting messages is public key encryption. This technology requires every participant to have a pair of "keys." The public key is shared over the Internet. The other key is private. Messages encrypted with the public key can be unencrypted only by the private key. The patient, for example, can send a message to the therapist by encrypting it with the therapist's public key so that only the therapist can unencrypt it with his or her private key. Although this method may seem quite secure, Mandl et al. note that authenticated persons commit most breaches of confidentiality of electronic data. They believe that further study is needed to provide a framework for developing policies, educational programs, and effective legislation.

File Transfer Protocol

One of the major uses of the Internet is the exchange or transfer of files. The **file transfer protocol (FTP)** is a way of sharing files. For many organizations, moving files from one organization, computer, or LAN to another is critical for business. For example, moving information on a patient's history and physical examination, an X-ray, or a client file from one computer to another facilitates communication among health care providers.

The word "transfer" in the acronym FTP is not entirely correct. Files do not actually transfer. They copy. In FTP one computer reads the contents of a file over the network and the other computer "listens" (Dern, 1994). The other computer then puts what it "hears" into a file on the hard drive. In this format, the receiver is then able to read the file and make changes to it or print it.

To use FTP, both the sending and receiving computers must have FTP available. To use FTP, it's necessary to know the address of the site where the file resides. Internet protocol (IP) is an address that consists of a series of numbers such as 234.56.789.01. Newer tools available on Internet navigators provide look-up of addresses that may appear as names or icons and transfer files quite easily. After the user accesses the site, a user ID and password are needed to get to the files. Sometimes a site requires a specific user ID; at other times, the word "anonymous" is the user ID. When entering the site, the user must know where the file resides. Directories are available, and decisions must be made regarding the type of transfer mode (binary, ASCII, or Auto Detect).

USENET

USENET newsgroups are online discussion groups that store messages in a news server, which the users view via a browser. Messages appear that everyone can see *(Fig. 11.1)*. Messages are not distributed to individual mailboxes, as they are with a listserv (Carlton & Miller, 1999). Dern (1994, p. 195) states that "if e-mail is the telephone and CB radio of the Internet, the USENET is its bulletin board, its supermarket tabloid, classified ad . . . and collective unconsciousness." USENET is a world-

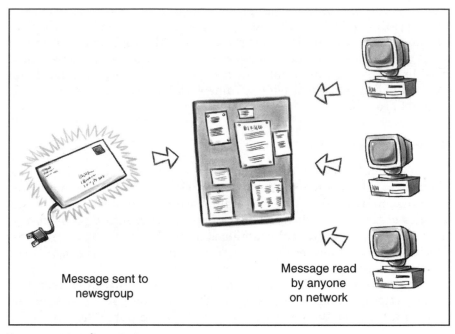

Message sent to
newsgroup

Message read
by anyone
on network

FIGURE 11.1 ▶ USENET newsgroups and bulletin boards.

wide community of **bulletin board services (BBSs)** closely associated with the Internet and the Internet community. Postings and comments to USENET groups pass among thousands of machines. According to Enzer (1999), only about half of all USENET machines are on the Internet. BBSs are organized discussions under a set of broad headings called "newsgroups" that allow the user to read and post messages (Tietze & Huber, 1995). An example is the occupational therapy newsgroup misc.health.therapy.occupational organized by Deja News, an Internet discussion site administrator (http://www.dejanews.com/). Characteristics of USENETs include handling short postings, sharing information but not rumors, and incorporating environments void of advertising. Users can post questions, answer questions, participate in discussions, learn information, retrieve or download programs, and find out about resources. More than 10,000 USENET newsgroups are available internationally, and many more are carried regionally or locally (Bull et al., 1997).

Access to BBSs is universal, so even if the topic is professional, anyone may participate. Thus, one is just as likely to find a member of the public, perhaps currently under treatment, posting a question about his or her therapy, as it is to find clinicians discussing treatment options among themselves. One of the problems with BBSs is the time and effort required to read the many messages posted every day. Therefore, the privacy and security of a listserv can be very attractive.

Listservs

Another type of e-mail discussion group is a listserv. **Listservs** differ from BBSs in that they are e-mail subscription lists maintained on a server distributing messages to members of a group. The listserv mailing program copies and sends all e-mail messages to subscribers *(Fig. 11.2)*. Other names for listservs are "discussion groups" and "mailing lists." Listservs offer information on thousands of topics. Liszt (http://www.liszt.com) produces one directory of listservs. Types of lists include mental health, patient safety, suicide prevention, occupational therapy, and nursing, among thousands of others. Be aware that just as people change their address by moving, so do listservs. In addition, listservs may cease to exist. Listservs may be moderated or unmoderated.

To subscribe to a listserv, the user must e-mail the listserv to request a subscription. Generally, an e-mail client is used, with the To: portion of the header addressed to the listserv (e.g., To: list@sailnet.com). Usually the subject line remains blank. In the body of the message, the subscriber usually types in the message "sub," "subscribe," or "join," followed by the first and last names or e-mail address (e.g., SUBSCRIBE

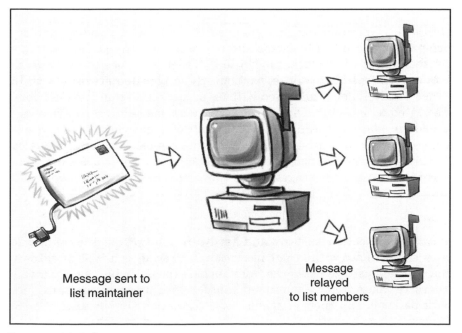

Message sent to
list maintainer

Message
relayed
to list members

FIGURE 11.2 ▶ Listservs.

macgregor-list James Leja or JOIN macgregor-list leja@wmich.edu). After that, the subscriber receives a message from the listserv confirming the subscription and providing information on useful commands. Sometimes the user is asked to confirm the request to join by replying to the message, whereas other listservs begin sending messages without confirmation. All subscribers see everything submitted, so it is advisable to be courteous with messages. If listserv messages fill a mailbox and are not retrieved, the subscriber may be dropped from the listserv.

Chat Rooms

Chat rooms are a synchronous service of the Web. Rather than responding to delayed e-mail and USENET postings, practitioners can engage in real-time conversations with their colleagues in chat rooms. Chat groups are online meetings where a number of self-helpers all log in to the same online "room" at the same time to exchange typed messages. Most self-help chat groups are found on the commercial services and meet at regularly scheduled times. On some commercial services, any member can start a chat group on any topic at any time. Chat groups are also sometimes called "live chat" or "real-time" meetings (Ferguson, 1996). Some health-related chat rooms focus on family issues, medicine and health, self-help, social issues, and women's health.

Security on the Internet

Electronic communication has changed the way health and human service providers conduct business and has created many issues related to the security of client data. Since the Internet is an open environment, data are susceptible to abuse, particularly in private networks with Internet access. If one is affiliated with an organization that uses networks associated with the Internet, it is likely that some security measures are already in place. According to Hebda and colleagues (1998), at least 20 percent of all organizations with an Internet connection have had a security breach. To secure access to private networks, **gateways** exist to intercept and inspect messages before they enter the private network.

Firewalls

Gateways are both a software and hardware solution used to connect local area networks with larger networks. A **firewall** is a type of gateway that protects private networks from hackers (people who secretly invade others' computers and examine or tamper with programs or data), network damage, and theft or misuse of information (Hebda et al., 1998). Firewalls screen traffic and allow only approved transactions to pass through them and restrict access to other systems or sensitive areas such as client information, payroll, or personnel data. Multiple firewalls increase protection.

Security Policies

Gateways and firewalls are not sufficient security to protect automated data. Other security measures are organizational in nature and require policies that are known and adhered to by all users. Hebda et al. (1998, p. 64), citing Leinfuss (1996) and Smith and Kallman (1996), identified a number of areas that should be addressed through policies. They include (1) the legal right of the organization to read employee e-mail unless otherwise stated; (2) the use of encryption; (3) obtaining consent from employees before transmitting employee data or photographs; (4) establishment of guidelines regarding intellectual property ownership; (5) a clear delineation of what the organization regards as ideas and images that are offensive or inappropriate; (6) what is acceptable Internet use in the workplace; (7) what constitutes plagiarism; and (8) a form of acknowledgment that the employee has received the policies.

Some breaches of security and confidentiality, despite policies, are unintentional. Because computers link offices and organizations, having access to a computer may also allow access to records or sensitive data. Dale Miller, a computer consultant with Irongate, Inc., believes that the most serious threat to data security isn't a computer hacker, but rather the scrap of paper in the desk drawer with the password that allows access to the computer and data (Tabar, 1997). Miller states that there are three commonsense things that can be done to minimize unauthorized viewing of data: (1) users should position computer monitors so that the screen cannot be seen by nonauthorized personnel; (2) anyone coming from an outside firm to repair computers should be required to sign a confidentiality statement; and (3) printouts should be destroyed. Miller is quoted as saying that "People perceive the risk [to security] as being the transmission of data, but the real risk is actually at the ends—where people are printing, sharing passwords, or talking about information in the elevator" (Tabar, 1997).

Intranet

Whereas the Internet allows users to read files, listen to music, and view graphics from remote locations across the world, the **intranet** is an in-house communications network. The intranet uses Internet technologies on an internal computer network. The Web model allows workers across an organization to create and maintain locally their own information services. Information resources need no longer be centralized within an information services department. Companies such as Pharmacia-Upjohn, a pharmaceutical firm with offices located throughout the world, can maintain policy manuals, phone books, and internal databases for their own use. Online manuals and information packets are maintained and updated easily. Coiera (1997) foresees intranets having the potential to change the model by which information is distributed. "In the past it was common for the author of a document to have to arrange for its distribution to all those who had an interest in it, either in paper or electronic form. In the Web model, it is possible for the author of information to simply make it available on a network, and place the onus on those with an interest to retrieve it" (p. 253).

WORLD WIDE WEB (WEB)

The **World Wide Web (Web)** is the fastest-growing and most dynamic feature of the Internet. In much the same way that fax services overlay the telephone system, the Web functions on top of the Internet's transport system. Hughes (1993) describes the Web as a "wide-area hypermedia information retrieval initiative aiming to give universal access to a large universe of documents." The Web is an easy-to-use method of accessing different kinds of information from just about anywhere in the world. It operates in a graphical environment and offers pictures, sound, animation, and video in addition to the display of textual information. The Web uses hypertext or hyperlinks to travel within and among Web-based media. **Hypertext** is essentially the same as the text in a book except that it contains connections within the text to other documents. Dern (1994) refers to this concept as a kind of "cosmic Chutes and Ladders." Generally, hypertext is set apart from regular text by a change of color or by underlining. The Web also uses **hypermedia** that is different from hypertext in that it contains links not only to other text, but also to other media such as sounds, images, and movies. Images themselves can take on the characteristic of a hyperlink. Generally, the user can discriminate regular text and images from hypertext and hypermedia by the change of appearance of the mouse arrow to a hand with a pointing finger or whatever configuration is set by the user when text and images are passed over the hyperlink.

How the Web Works

For most users, their window onto the Web is provided by a program called a **browser**. A Web browser is an application used to access the Web and use its functionality (Gee, 1997). Most browsers have forward, backward, reload, and stop buttons. **Bookmarks** enable the user to mark frequently visited sites for rapid access in the future. When one uses a popular Web browser (e.g., Netscape or Microsoft Internet Explorer) to view a Web page, hypertext such as "Healthcare Informatics" may appear. When the user selects or clicks on the hypertext, the computer connects to another computer specified by a network address somewhere on the Internet and asks that computer's Web server for "Healthcare Informatics." The server responds and sends text and other media to the user's screen.

The language used by Web clients and servers to communicate with one another is called the **HyperText Transmission Protocol (http)**. The letters "http" are the first four letters appearing in the Netsite or Address line usually found in the top banner portion of both Netscape and Microsoft Internet Explorer. For creating and recognizing hypermedia documents, one of the standard Web languages is **HyperText Markup Language (HTML)**; however, Web languages are evolving, and new versions appear constantly. Web documents are basic **ASCII (American Standard Code for Information Interchange)** files with formatting codes containing information about the layout (document titles, paragraphs, colors, etc.) and hyperlinks.

HTML uses **uniform resource locators (URLs)** to symbolize hyperlinks. The part of the URL before the two slashes specifies the method of access, such as http or ftp. The second portion of the address is commonly the address on the computer where the data are located. For example, the URL for F. A. Davis Company is http://www.fadavis.com, where http is the method of access, www.fadavis is the address, and com represents a commercial or business site.

The development of **plug-in** or helper **programs** adds to the repertoire of browsers. Plug-ins are usually small pieces of software developed by people other than the publishers of the software with which the plug-ins work. Examples of plug-ins include audio and video players in addition to animation software. The programming languages for plug-ins are usually JavaScript, C++, or ActiveX. Java, developed by Sun Microsystems, enables the display of moving text, animations, and music on Web pages.

Search Engines

Search engines are critical for helping users locate information on the Web. According to the "Spider's Apprentice" site maintained for Monash Information Systems (Barlow, 1999), search engines use software "robots," "crawlers," "worms," or "spiders" to query the Web. Webcrawler is an example of a search engine that uses a spider. These software programs are constantly at work on the Internet, acquiring and updating databases. Sparks and Rizzolo (1998, p. 167) note that the Lycos search tool received its name from the Latin word "Lycosidae," the "name for a family of large active ground spiders that catch their prey by pursuit, rather than in a web." Lycosidae are nocturnal and noted for their great running speed.

When a question or query is entered at the search engine site, the query is checked against the keyword indices of the search engine. The two primary methods of text searching are the keyword and the concept. Keyword searches are probably the most common method used by search engines to query and retrieve text. According to Barlow (1999), search engines pull out and index words believed to be important. Words that appear at the top of the document or that are repeated often throughout the document are perceived by the search engine as important.

Three parts make up the search engine: a search interface, a database or index, and a spider (robot, worm, or crawler). The spider travels over the Internet to various sites and then places the information in the database or index. When a user enters a query into the search engine, the program checks for matches, formatting them into a results list and displaying the results for the user. The only humans involved in this process are the programmers who wrote the programs for the spider, database, and search algorithm. The program determines the contents of the database.

Metasearching is a powerful way to search the Internet for specific information. Instead of just searching one database, like Lycos, metasearch engines query multiple search services. One example of a metasearch engine is MetaCrawler. After the user inputs a query, MetaCrawler sends it to several Web search engines including Lycos, Infoseek, Excite, WebCrawler, AltaVista, and Yahoo!, among others. Metasearch engines perform searches in one of two ways. They can search specific search engines in the order the user selects, such as with the metasearch engine Starting Point, or they can perform searches using several tools simultaneously, eliminating redundant hits, as does MetaCrawler.

The best metasearch engines tell the user how many results came from each Web search engine, sort the results, remove duplicates, and indicate the Web search engine from which the results came. The format of the response varies, but the result is that the user has the most relevant "hits" from a number of Web search engines with only one request. Useful features of the metasearch engine include the ability to limit the search geographically or by domain (e.g., edu, com, gov), the choice of speed or a comprehensive parallel search, and the ability to limit the retrieval time (Sparks & Rizollo, 1998).

Another method of searching the Web is a **subject directory**. Yahoo! is one of the earliest subject directories and the largest, with nearly a million entries. Two major differences exist between a subject directory and a Web search engine. First, in subject directories, entries are selected by human beings; therefore, the resulting database is smaller and more selective (Rollason, 1997). Second, subject directories are arranged by subject or category, adding another layer of organization. In general, subject directories work best when locating broad categories of information—the area where Web search engines fail. Subject directories are so important that they have been included in most of the major Web search engines *(Table 11.1)*.

TABLE 11.1 ▶ **MAJOR SEARCH AND METASEARCH TOOLS AND SUBJECT DIRECTORIES**

Search Tool	Uniform Resource Locator
AltaVista	http://www.altavista.digital.com
Excite	http://www.excite.com
Hotbot	http://www.hotbot.com
InfoSeek	http://www.infoseek.com
Lycos	http://www.lycos.com
Northern Light	http://www.northernlight.com
Metasearch Tools	**Uniform Resource Locator**
Profusion	http://www.profusion.com
Inference Find	http://www.wisdomdog.com
Cyber411	http://www.cyber411.com
Dogpile	http://www.dogpile.com
Metafind	http://www.metafind.com
Highway61	http://www.highway61.com
Subject Directories	**Uniform Resource Locator**
Yahoo!	http://www.yahoo.com
Virtual Library	http://www.virtuallibrary.com
Looksmart	http://www.looksmart.com
Magellan	http://www.magellan.com

Evaluating Web Sites

The Web has grown rapidly since its inception. Documents published on the Web reach thousands of viewers and are relatively easy and inexpensive to create. Anyone with access to the Web can create a personal site and include information believed to be pertinent. Many Web sites are commercial ventures, providing an opportunity to view the company's wares; others are personal Web sites reflecting the personality and biases of the author. Web sites are not censored, evaluated for content, or peer reviewed. Anyone can publish anything on the Web. The information within the site reflects the opinion of the developer, who also assumes responsibility for the content and accuracy of the site. Because the content of the Web is unmonitored, users must carefully evaluate Web-based information. Kapoun (1998) suggests five criteria for **Web site evaluation**: accuracy, authority, objectivity, currency, and coverage of the site.

When evaluating the accuracy of Web documents, it is important to consider if the information is accurate, reliable, and free from error because Web standards to ensure accuracy are not fully developed. To determine accuracy, the contents of the site must be evaluated in light of other documentation on the subject. The Web is only one source of information and can be very useful for researching certain topics. However, to research a topic thoroughly, a variety of both Web and non-Web sources is needed. The use of editors and fact checkers for the Web site increase confidence that the material is accurate, but they cannot be the sole indicators of correctness.

To determine the authority of a document, look for the credentials of the author and note the publisher. The author should include an e-mail address, telephone number, or physical address. An important question to consider is, "Do the credentials of the author qualify him or her to fulfill the purpose of the document?" Check the domain (gov, edu, com, mil, org) of the document. How reputable is the publisher? Keep in mind that there is a distinction between the Webmaster, the person maintaining the site, and the author of the document or site. It is often difficult to determine the authorship of Web sources. If the author's name is listed, the qualifications frequently are absent and the publisher's identity is often not indicated.

Regarding objectivity, it is necessary to determine the goals and objectives of the site. The goals and aims of persons or groups presenting the material often are not clearly stated. Is the information presented with a minimum of bias? To what extent is the information trying to sway the opinion of the audience? Also, note the amount of detail in the information and the opinions, if any, expressed by the author.

Currency of a site is important if the information needed must be up to date. Treatment- or drug-related information may be most valuable when it is current. Look for both publication and update dates. Often the date of the last update is given somewhere on the page, usually near the bottom. Dead links indicate neglect, whereas a well-maintained site updates links regularly.

When examining the coverage of the Web document, decide whether complete viewing of the information requires a special browser or the payment of a fee. Software requirements and fees limit access to the information. Are the topics at the site explored in depth or is the information introductory or shallow? Assess whether the links are relevant to the site's subject. The quality of pages linked to the original (home) page may vary. A high-quality home page may be linked with a poor-quality page. Determine if the presented information is cited. Evaluate the subject matter's presentation. Is it presented solely through images or are the images accompanied by text?

An additional challenge when evaluating coverage concerns the proliferation of marketing-oriented Web pages. These sites blend entertainment, information, and advertising. In print sources there is usually a clear distinction between advertising and information, but on the Web this distinction is easily blurred. The reader must determine if advertising and information are being supplied by the same person or organization. If so, advertising is likely to bias the information.

Evaluation of Web sites is not an easy task, as information is often missing or difficult to find. Establishing an evaluation procedure helps the professional determine the usefulness of Web information (Alexander & Tate, 1996). The first step in an evaluation procedure is to identify the type of page presented. Common types are entertainment, business, marketing, reference, informational, news, advocacy, and personal. The second step is to use a checklist to evaluate the site according to the five criteria of accuracy, authority, objectivity, currency, and coverage. Based on the outcome of the checklist, the third step is to determine the overall quality of the page. A site may not meet all of the criteria, but the more "yes" answers on the checklist, the higher the quality of the site.

Development of Web evaluation techniques is just beginning. Technology is outpacing the ability to create standards and guidelines for evaluation. Establishing evaluation procedures is an ongoing process.

Using the Web for Professional Purposes

Information on the Web is useful to the healthcare professional for developing professional life and practice, obtaining disease-oriented information, and delivering healthcare information to the consumer. Professional life and practice are enhanced by professional organization sites informing members and nonmembers of the organization's activities, publications, and personnel information. Professional sites often link with organizations providing online continuing education for a nominal fee and employment opportunities. The major publishers of healthcare information provide multipurpose sites including electronic journals, abstracts, publication archives, current-interest information, and chat rooms for discussions with authors or for discussions about current issues affecting the profession. Professional listservs keep practitioners in contact with colleagues of similar interest around the world.

Disease information from lay to professional levels is available for both common and rare diseases. Information about the latest research on specific diseases may take as long as 1 to 2 years for publication in print media. On the Web, research information can be updated daily. National disease-specific associations, such as the American Cancer Society, the American Diabetes Forum, and the National Alliance for the Mentally Ill maintain excellent informational sites, as do some support groups. Universities and teaching hospitals also maintain sites with superb information about specific diseases. One must always evaluate the sites according the five evaluation criteria to determine the validity of the information.

The Internet has given consumers access to a wide range of health information. One of the main impacts of the Web on the consumer and practitioner is the increased possibility for patients to act as their own best advocates. But the quantity of information available on the Web is immense. Hafner (1998) states that more than 10,000 sites with information from experts, amateurs, and quacks, coupled with instant accessibility, are bringing about a shift in the way doctors and patients interact. She goes on to say that at its best, the Internet transforms the doctor-patient relationship into a partnership that saves lives. At its worst, information found online is misleading or inaccurate.

In 1998 an estimated 18 million adults surfed online for health information, ranking it as one of the top five subjects people search for, reports CyberDialogue, an Internet market research company in New York (Wynn, 1999). Hafner (1998) points out that two-thirds of the people who went online were seeking health information. Further, she indicates, 5 percent of these Web users found it very difficult to interpret and understand information they located on the Web. Sixty-seven percent of doctors stated that they had patients who came into the office with information they had found on the Internet, but only 12 percent of doctors referred patients to the Internet.

An example of a consumer-oriented medical site is Mediconsult.com, which claims to be the "Web destination that patients use most," with 14 million page requests in 1997 (Worldwide Nurse, 1998). This site provides patient-oriented health information, journal articles, and drug information, as well as interactive activities such as moderated patient support groups and scheduled live events. The posted information is reviewed for accuracy and pertinence to patients and their families. The language is jargon-free and understandable to anyone who visits the site.

Provider organizations are beginning to utilize consumers' interest in the Web. In 1997 Kaiser Permanente developed a pilot project providing its patients with a personal identification number (PIN) access and an online, nonurgent appointment-scheduling system. Kaiser Permanente patients can also search 30,000 pages of disease-specific information; participate in discussion groups; and send questions to a nurse, pharmacist, or specialist. Kaiser Permanente also has plans for an online pharmacy (Schneider, 1997).

The Comprehensive Health Enhancement Support System (CHESS) is a network of home health workstations maintained by the University of Wisconsin for people with AIDS, breast cancer, and other diseases. CHESS links patients to each other and to care providers, medical information libraries, and other resources (Essex, 1999).

Online systems are beginning to make the grand database of professional medicine accessible to everyone. Laypersons now have access to most of the same information professionals rely on. In this Information Age of healthcare, it is the health-active consumer, the concerned and supportive family caretaker, the neighborhood natural helper, the corporate wellness professional, and perhaps other key players yet to evolve, working in cooperation with a new generation of supportive health professionals, who will serve as the real primary practitioners, says Dr. Tom Ferguson (1996). According to Ferguson, preliminary studies suggest that online health systems can reduce costs while improving the quality of healthcare.

As advocates for patient health, practitioners are well advised to keep abreast of the information resources their patients are consulting. Directing Internet-savvy patients to excellent Web sites enhances patient teaching. Teaching patients how to evaluate Web sites increases their ability to access valid and reliable information.

COMMUNICATION TECHNOLOGIES

While the Internet has had tremendous influence on information processing in healthcare, other communication technologies are also influencing the industry. Newer miniature testing and monitoring machines are profoundly changing the delivery of healthcare. Portable electrocardiogram machines provide an immediate rhythm strip by simply resting the machine on the chest of the patient; no wires are required (Bayne, 1997). Blood analysis technology reduced to portable size analyzes blood gases, four electrolytes, hemoglobin and hematocrit, blood urea nitrogen, glucose, and calcium from a single drop of blood. A handheld magnetic resonance image (MRI) scanner that does not require radiation protection moves from place to place. Analyzing the human factors of advancing technology is an important role for the healthcare professional of the future.

Personal Digital Assistants and Palmtops

The popularity of **personal digital assistants (PDAs)** and palmtops is increasing in healthcare. A PDA is a specialized handheld device used primarily to keep appointments, calendars, addresses, and telephone numbers. Since the inception of the concept in 1993, when Apple Computer introduced the first PDA product, the Newton Message Pad, PDAs have expanded both in capability and in the number of manufacturers. PDAs like PalmPilot and Casio's Cassiopeia offer features that may be beneficial to healthcare providers. In addition to offering calendar, addressing, and note-taking functions, they come with modems, multimedia, voice recording, and e-mail functions. For example, DSM-IV or a medical English-Spanish dictionary is available for many PDAs. A company called 1ST STOP offers a full-featured, mobile record system that it says has the ability to generate a patient's history and physical exam record, progress notes, discharge summaries, referral request letters, and a database of 1200 medications. For the PalmPilot, there are many commercial, freeware, and shareware healthcare-related programs that include drug interaction databases, medical mathpads, and the Folstein Mini Mental Status Exam. Again, the user must decide what applications and functions are desirable.

Voice Recognition

Voice recognition is not a new idea. It has been available in a limited form since the mid-1980s. The principal method of voice recognition compares digital patterns of single words spoken by the person with stored digital copies of words to come up with the best match (Roe, 1994).

The types of speech recognition technologies are numerous. Speaker-dependent voice recognition requires users to participate in fairly extensive exercises to train the computer to develop a voice profile that attempts to match the user's voice synthesizations (Dunn, 1995). Another type, speaker-independent voice recognition, does not require the user to go through extensive training; the user can begin to use the software once it is installed. Discrete speech input requires the user to pause between every word. Padilla (1997) states that despite these pauses, users can achieve a rate of over 80 words per minute. Another type of speech input is continuous speech, which allows the user to speak in fluid sentences that sound more natural. Finally, natural speech, still in the developmental stages, is the ultimate in voice recognition, allowing users to talk to their computers in no specific manner and have the computer understand. The most important aspect of voice recognition is accuracy. If the software is unable to translate what is said correctly, it is of no value.

In an article appearing in the October 20, 1998, issue of *PC Magazine* on what to look for in speech recognition programs, the editors stated that editing and formatting, application integration, and command and control are critical components. They reviewed a number of products, including Dragon Naturally Speaking and IBM's ViaVoice, and reported the results of some of the ways in which the various programs interpreted sample phrases. For example, when the tester said "cold training and mop-up" the program heard "college training in Moscow" (wysiwyg:// 175/http://www.zdnet.com/pcmag/features/speech98/sayagain.html). It's no wonder that Jesse Berst, editorial director at the ZDNet AnchorDesk, in the April 1, 1999, issue, remained skeptical about the use of speech software as a replacement for the mouse or the keyboard at this time.

SUMMARY

The use of electronic communications in health and human service practices continues to grow. More and more healthcare professionals are communicating with their patients and colleagues, receiving diagnostic information, keeping up to date, and providing patient teaching through the use of technology. The development of the Internet, with its protocols for e-mail, FTP, USENET, listservs, chat groups, and the use of organizational intranets, enables practitioners to communicate quickly and easily with each other. The World Wide Web, with its powerful information search engines, has made a profound impact on how basic information and new knowledge obtained through research are disseminated. Security of the information continues to be an issue, but hardware and software technology such as firewalls and thoughtful, well-understood personnel policies have increased the protection of the information. New communication technologies such as PDAs and voice recognition systems promise to streamline both access to information and input of information at the point of care. Although it is not always necessary to understand the details of the technologies' use—and these continue to evolve—it is necessary to understand their potential for improving local, regional, national, and global health.

▶ LEARNING EXERCISES

1. Subscribe to at least one listserv in your profession and monitor the conversations for 2 weeks. Identify one topic among the conversations that seems particularly relevant to your profession.
2. Using a search engine of your choosing, locate four Web sites related to your profession and critique them, using the criteria provided in this chapter.
3. Use a second search engine to search as above. What different sites did you find?
4. Use e-mail to communicate with a professional in your field outside of your institution. How will you find such a person?
5. Interview a health and human services professional and see how he or she uses electronic communications at work.
6. Determine if your organization has a policy regarding the use of electronic media. How does your organization deal with confidentiality, privacy, and other ethical issues related to the use of electronic communications?
7. Select a topic of interest and develop a two-page paper using resources you found on the Web.

References

Alexander, J. A., & Tate, M. (1996). *Web evaluation power point presentation* [Online]. Available: http://www.science.widener.edu/~withers/alaslides [1999, July 10].

Barlow, L. (1999). *How search engines work. The Spider's apprentice* [Online]. Available: http://www.monash.com/spidap4.html [1999, July 10].

Bayne, C. G. (1997). Pocket-sized medicine: New POC technologies. *Nursing Management, 28*(8), 30–32.

Berst, J. (1999, April 1). *What they're not telling you about speech recognition. Jesse Berst's AnchorDesk* [Online]. Available: http://www.zdnet.com/anchordesk/story/story_3247.html.

Bull, G., Bull, G., & Sigmon, T. (1997). Internet discussion groups. *Learning and Leading with Technology, 25*(3), 12–17.

Carlton, K. H., & Miller, P. A. (1999). Asynchronous communication technology tools in practice—future and current uses. *Computers in Nursing, 17*(4), 162–165.

Coiera, E. (1997). *Guide to medical informatics, the Internet and telemedicine.* Oxford: Alden Press.

Dern, D. (1994). *The Internet guide for new users.* New York: McGraw-Hill.

Dunn, J. (1995, November 27). Speech recognition solutions: Speaking your mind. *Infoworld, 17*(48), 28–30.

Enzer, M. (1999). Glossary of Internet terms. At http://matisse.net/files/glossary.htm.

Essex, D. (1999, February). Life line. *Healthcare Informatics,* 120.

Ferguson, T. (1996). *Health online.* Reading, MA: Addison-Wesley.

Gee, P. M. (1997). The Internet: A home care nursing clinical resource. *Home Healthcare Nurse, 15*(2), 115–121.

Hafner, K. (1998, July 9). Can the Internet cure the common cold? *The New York Times,* p. G1.

Hebda, T., Czar, P., & Mascara, C. (1998*). Handbook of informatics for nurses and health care professionals.* Menlo Park, CA: Addison-Wesley.

Hughes, K. (1993). *Entering the World-Wide Web: A guide to cyberspace* [Online]. Available: http://www.hcc.hawaii.edu/guide/www.guide.html#2 [1999, July 12].

Jones telecommunications and multimedia encyclopedia.(1999) [Online]. Available: http://www.digitalcentury.com/encyclo/update/comp_hd.html [1999, July 12].

Kapoun, J. (1998). Teaching undergraduate Web evaluation. *College and Research Library News, 59*(7), 522–523.

Leinfuss, E. (1996). Policy over pricing. *Infoworld, 18*(24), 8.

Mandl, K., Kohane, I., & Brandt, A. (1998). Electronic patient–physician communication: Problems and promise. *Annals of Internal Medicine, 129,* 495–500.

Microsoft Press. (1991). *Computer dictionary.* Redmond, OR: Author.

Padilla, E. (1997, January 21). In Onken, M. *Voice recognition* [Online]. Available: http://cc.weber.edu/~itfm/hottopic/VOICEREC/Voicerec.htm#Definition [1999, July 13].

Roe, D. (1994). *Speech synthesis technology: Voice communication between humans and machines* (pp. 159–199). Washington, DC: National Academy of Sciences.

Rollason, D. H. (1997, March). The clinician's net: Internet services and indexes. *Physician Assistant,* 150–170.

Say that again???? (1998, October 20). *PC Magazine, 17*(17), .

Schneider, P. (1997, August). Patient informatics is growing. *Healthcare Informatics,* 26.

Smith, J. J., & Kallman, E. A. (1996). Managing the Net. *Beyond Computing, 5*(3), 14–15.

Sparks, S. M., & Rizzolo, M. A. (1998). World Wide Web search tools. *Image: Journal of Nursing Scholarship, 30*(2), 167–171.

Tabar, P. (1997). *The common sense of physician practice security. Informatics: News and trends* [Online]. Available: http://healthcare-informatics.com/issue/1997/09_97/n_t.htm.

Tappendorf, S. (1995). *ARPANET and beyond* [Online]. Available: http://clavin.music.uiuc.edu/sean/intrnet_history.html.

Tietze, M., & Huber, J. (1995). Electronic information retrieval in nursing. *Nursing Management, 26*(7), 36–42.

Worldwide Nurse. (1998). [Online]. Available: http://www.wwnurse.com [1999, July 14].

Wynn, P. (1999). Physicians leap into cyberspace. *Physicians Financial News, 17*(9), 14.

12

Telehealth

LYNNE M. PATZEK MILLER AND KATHLEEN M. YOUNG

LEARNING OBJECTIVES

By the end of this chapter, you will be able to:
▶ Define various types of telecommunications
▶ Discuss the advantages of telehealth
▶ Identify the equipment and technology used to support
  telecommunications

211

▶ Discuss the obstacles to telehealth
▶ Describe various applications of telehealth

Noticing that an 8-year-old second-grade boy in an inner-city school was flushed and listless during class, the teacher sent him to the school nurse's office to have his temperature taken. The boy described an extreme sore throat and an earache. His temperature was 102°F. The school file revealed that his single, working mother had no personal transportation, so she could not pick him up at school. The file also contained a signed permission for a medical consultation via the telecommunication system connecting the school and a university clinic. After the school connected with the clinic, the boy was examined electronically using an online stethoscope and otoscope (for the throat and ears). With the school nurse placing the instruments, the physician at the clinic was able to hear the heart and lung sounds and see the condition of the ears and throat. After making a diagnosis, the physician notified the family's pharmacy of the prescribed medication that the mother could pick up on her way home from work. The communication equipment between the school and the clinic provided a student in an underserved, inner-city school with a physician examination, timely diagnosis, and treatment that he might otherwise not have received.

A federal prisoner developed an irregular heartbeat requiring the expertise of a cardiologist. Rather than transport the prisoner to the cardiologist, requiring at least two guards and a driver, the infirmary at the prison connected electronically with the specialist at the university hospital. Using sophisticated telecommunications equipment, the specialist interviewed the patient and performed an electronic examination of his heart and lungs. The electrocardiogram (EKG) pattern obtained at the prison was faxed to the university, providing the physician with the information necessary to complete the examination. The physician then prescribed treatment and medication without the need for either the prisoner or the physician to travel. The long-distance examination provided safety for the prisoner and the public, an immediate examination by a specialist, and timely initiation of treatment.

A long-term diabetic uses a glucose meter to monitor his blood sugar level several times each day. The glucometer features easy-to-use, menu-driven screens that capture data and analyze options, including trending graphs and charts. The meter can be tailored to the individual, including diet and exercise factors. Once the man tests his blood glucose level and answers the lifestyle questions posed by the meter, the glucometer stores the readings and information. At the end of the day the patient attaches the glucometer to the telephone, and with a push of a button he faxes the readings to his physician's office. The physician analyzes the data and offers appropriate advice. The diabetic gets help without having to travel to see a physician, saving time and money. Problems are addressed before they worsen and before the patient ends up in the hospital.

Each of these scenarios is an example of the use of telecommunications technologies for the provision of long-distance clinical health care. The use of telecommunications in healthcare, also known as "telehealth," is also important in distance education and administration. The consulting firm Deloitte and Touche predicts that telecommunication in healthcare will be big business by 2002 (Edlin, 1999). Based on the 35 percent aggregate growth rate of 1997, the company estimates that there will be a $3 billion U.S. market in the new millennium.

TERMS RELATED TO TELEHEALTH

Chaffee (1999) and others offer the following definitions for telehealth concepts:

Asynchronous Transfer Mode (ATM): A high-speed data transmission link that can carry large amounts of data quickly. ATM works well when large sets of data such as magnetic resonance imaging (MRI) data need to be exchanged and discussed. The use of ATM is limited because of the high cost, lack of availability, and lack of standards.

Bandwidth: The amount of digital information that can be sent through a system or channel (Coiera, 1997, p. 210). It is similar to the capacity of a pipe to carry water: the larger the pipe, the more water transported. Inexpensive telephone lines have a narrow bandwidth and do not transmit video images. Broad-bandwidth networks transmit moving images but are costly.

Integrated Service Digital Network (ISDN): A method of transmission through telephone lines. ISDN lines do not have the bandwidth of SMDS lines, but they do have greater capacity than plain old telephone service (POTS), although POTS is rapidly gaining the capacity of ISDN lines. ISDN lines can also be leased at a fixed monthly rate. They support medical imaging, database sharing, desktop videoconferencing, and access to the Internet.

Switched Multimegabit Data Service (SMDS): An option for high-speed transmission. SMDS is also known as "T1 lines." These are high-speed telephone lines that are leased monthly at a fixed rate. They are used to transmit high-quality, full-motion video.

Telecommunications: Transmission of information from one site to another in the form of signs, signals, words, or pictures by cable, radio, or other systems. Examples include telephone calls, cable television programming, facsimile transmissions, satellite paging systems, and e-mail.

Teleconferencing: The use of audio, and possibly video, equipment at different locations to carry out telehealth applications (Hebda et al., 1998, p. 249). Teleconferencing is often accomplished through videoconferencing and desktop videoconferencing (DTV). Videoconferencing, using sounds and images, saves travel time and reduces costs, encouraging people to meet more frequently. DTV is a synchronous, or real-time, encounter that uses a specially equipped personal computer with a telephone line hookup to allow people to meet face-to-face and/or view papers and images simultaneously (Hebda et al., 1998, p. 250). DTV may not contain the picture resolution or speed of transmission required for telemedicine, such as interpretation of diagnostic images, diagnosis of dermatological conditions, or analysis of a patient's movements, but it is adequate for administrative meetings.

Telehealth: Use of telecommunications equipment and communications networks to transfer healthcare information between participants at different locations. It provides long-distance clinical healthcare, patient and professional education, and health administration. It encompasses telemedicine and telenursing, as well as a broad spectrum of information technologies for healthcare providers and consumers. Equipment includes computers, telephones, video monitors, and telecommunications networks connecting two or more sites.

Telehealth systems permit the provision of care in situations where a face-to-face meeting between patient and provider may be impossible or costly. Telehealth provides healthcare to underserved communities and professional education to wide geographic areas.

Telemedicine, telenursing, teleradiology, telepathology, teleoncology, teledermatology, etc.: Subsets of telehealth. Telehealth focuses on practicing healthcare in specific disciplines through the use of a telecommunications system. Most practitioners already use telecommunications: telephones and fax machines.

Telepresence: The virtual (not actual) presence of an individual in a room. Making a student at a distant site feel that he or she is in the actual presence of an instructor is important in distance education. Telepresence helps patients feel that they are in the company of a specialist in a telehealth consultation. Telepresence can also combine robotics and virtual reality to allow a surgeon equipped with special gloves and proper video and audio equipment to manipulate surgical instruments at a remote site. The European Institute of Telesurgery in Strasbourg, France, conducts teletraining sessions incorporating multimedia demonstrations, medical image exchange, and real-time conferencing among experts in different countries on actual cases. Over 4000 surgeons have participated in training at the institute. This training provides a global way for surgeons to reduce the learning curve, discover new procedures, and consult with peers. The teleconferencing network currently links more than 30 medical centers in Europe, North America, and Japan (Tabar, 1999).

HISTORICAL PERSPECTIVE ON TELEHEALTH

Telehealth, in its earliest stages, involved physicians using the telephone to contact other physicians for consultation in interpreting clinical findings, determining a diagnosis, and formulating a treatment plan.

Electronic signaling technology, including two-way radios and closed-circuit television, in use since 1955, were the next step toward telehealth (*What Is Telemedicine*, 1999). However, some of the most aggressive uses of telehealth occurred because of the technological advances made at the National Aeronautics and Space Administration (NASA) (Hebda et al., 1998, p. 250). NASA provided international telemedicine consultations for victims following the Armenian earthquake in 1989 and currently is researching the process of feeding images from the battlefield to physicians in a field hospital behind the lines for improved treatment of the wounded.

Some early telehealth programs are the following:

- In 1955 the Nebraska Medical Center Psychiatric Institute employed a two-way closed-circuit television system using a microwave technology link with the Norfolk State Hospital 112 miles away for education, consultation, and interaction between the specialists and general practitioners. In 1971 they expanded their services to include the Omaha Veterans' Administration (VA) Hospital and two other VA institutions (House & Roberts, 1977).
- In the 1960s the NASA space program, using a satellite system, transmitted the vital signs of the astronauts from the spacecraft and space suits to physicians monitoring them at the NASA Space Center (Bashshur & Lovett, 1977).
- In 1967, responding to a need at the Logan International Airport, Massachusetts General Hospital (MGH) used a two-way microwave technology system to provide emergency care and medical attention to the travelers and employees at the airport. Nurses were available 24 hours a day to evaluate patients. Using electronic transmission equipment, the nurses were able to send assessment findings, x-ray and microscope images, EKG readings, vital signs, and other pertinent data to an MGH physician. A diagnosis was then made and treatment instituted (Murphy & Bird, 1974).
- In 1971 the National Library of Medicine at Lister Hill National Center for Biomedical Communications, Bethesda, MD, selected 26 sites in Alaska and established a two-way audio and satellite video system to improve the communication and quality of healthcare to the rural villages. An evaluation of the Alaska ATS-6 Satellite Biomedical Demonstration revealed that the satellite system was "workable" and could be used in various locations for most medical problems except emergencies. The ATS-6 Satellite project has expanded and is still in use (Foote et al., 1976).
- In 1972 the Indian Health Service, the Department of Health, Education, and Welfare, and NASA conceived and engineered a

program to provide healthcare on the Papago Indian reservation. Two Indian paramedics staffed a van with a two-way microwave and audio transmission system and a variety of medical instruments, including EKG and x-ray equipment. Linking the system to a public health hospital and other hospitals and specialists provided healthcare to the natives of the reservation (Bashshur, 1980).

- Funded by grants from the federal government, telemedicine projects flourished in the 1980s. The purpose of much of this early research was to determine whether telehealth would work. Most of the projects did demonstrate that telehealth worked but that it was very expensive. When the grant monies were exhausted, the telehealth initiatives ceased because they were not solvent (Chaffee, 1999). Lack of federal grants caused a decline in the use of and research for telehealth.

- Interest in telehealth surged again in the 1990s as the healthcare delivery system focused on reducing costs while increasing quality of care and access. Passage of Georgia's Distance Learning and Telemedicine Act of 1992 resulted in a windfall of $50 million from telephone company overearnings. Rather than refund the money to consumers, legislators created a fund to finance telecommunications projects in medicine and education. The project designers created a full-service system providing a comprehensive range of clinical and consultative services to all residents of the state through a hub-and-spoke network. The plan consists of several tertiary-care centers and a set of secondary hubs at medical centers throughout the state. Each hub, in turn, serves several remote sites. The system enables connectivity throughout the network. The Center for Telemedicine at the Medical College of Georgia provides overall coordination, implementation, and oversight (Adams & Grigsby, 1995).

- In 1995 the University of Texas–Galveston (UTG) initiated an interactive telehealth program that has been used for over 2500 remote consultations a year. Funded by the Rural Health Project, consultations include all specialty services utilizing modern audio and visual technology. UTG is the largest telemedicine facility in the nation (Auton, 1999).

- In 1989, 16 states were active in telemedicine development (Lipson & Henderson, 1996). Just 9 years later, in 1998, the federal government administered 41 telehealth and telemedicine grants in 29 states totaling more than $13.6 million (Office for the Advancement of Telehealth Services, 1999). Some states, particularly Georgia, Kansas, Texas, South Dakota, and Louisiana, have well-developed programs. Policy actions taken by the states in support of telehealth differ considerably. They include planning and coordination, development of networks, program development, funding, building a telecommunications infrastructure for telehealth, and providing regulatory support and clarification. A wide array of funding sources has been used, including state tax dollars and state-earmarked federal monies and regulatory judgments. The level of funding by the states has also varied, ranging from less than $100,000 to millions of dollars. Efforts to develop telehealth facilities appear likely to continue in order to improve access to health care.

The passage of the Telecommunications Act of 1995, which allows vendors of cable and telephone services to compete in each other's markets, removed a major barrier to telehealth (Schneider, 1996). The Snowe-Rockefeller Amendment (1997) requires telecommunications carriers to offer services to rural health providers at rates comparable to those charged in urban areas so that affordable healthcare may be available to rural residents. The federal government is again investing considerable research funds in the development of telehealth projects. Federal government agencies, including the Department of Defense, the Department of Health and Human Services, NASA, and the Department of Commerce, are devoting considerable resources to exploring the uses of telehealth. Global initiatives are also expanding with the use of telehealth to serve sparsely populated regions in Australia and Canada (Telemedicine Research Center, 1996).

TYPES OF TECHNOLOGY

Two different kinds of technology make up most of the telehealth applications in use today (Brown, 1999). The first, called **store and forward**, is used for transferring digital images from one location to another. A digital image is taken using a digital camera, stored, and then sent to another location. This method is typically used for nonemergency situations when a diagnosis or consultation may be made in the next 24–48 hours and sent back.

Store and forward is the most common application of telehealth today and is able to send x-rays, computed tomography (CT) scans, and MRI scans. Many radiologists are installing teleradiology equipment in their homes, so that radiology images are sent directly to them for diagnosis, avoiding the need for off-hours trips to a hospital or clinic. Pathologists and dermatologists also send digital images using store and forward applications.

The other widely-used technology, **two-way interactive television (IATV)**, is used when a consultation between the patient, primary care provider, and specialist is necessary. Videoconferencing equipment at both locations, typically an urban and a rural location, allows a real-time consultation to take place. Videoconferencing is also useful for administrative meetings, allowing the participants to communicate across distances without traveling from their office buildings. Videoconferencing is an appealing concept also used for distance learning.

Both types of technology are used in three areas comprising telehealth initiatives: clinical, academic, and administrative. Each of these areas benefits from the improved outcomes and lower cost of telecommunications technology.

CLINICAL INITIATIVES

Telehealth is applicable to a broad range of clinical initiatives encompassing healthcare for remote geographic areas, schools, prisons, emergency medicine, and home care. The applications vary greatly and include client monitoring, diagnostic evaluations, and image transmission for diagnosis and research. Sophisticated equipment is not always necessary. Some applications are highly technical, whereas others utilize very simple technology. Telecommunications is not an end in itself but a means to an end, which is to break down obstacles to care.

Rural Telehealth

Providing healthcare to rural and remote geographic locations is one of the most common applications of telehealth. The use of telecommunications in rural healthcare improves access to care and eliminates the barrier of distance. Historically, rural America has always had a difficult time providing healthcare to its residents (Puskin, 1992). For practitioners, the barrier of distance contributes to professional isolation, making it difficult to recruit and retain health professionals. Economically, lower incomes and more fragile economies make it difficult to sustain healthcare institutions. For patients, lack of access to the full range of healthcare affects the quality of life in the rural community. The lack of adequate technology infrastructure development is a key barrier to the diffusion of telecommunications in rural communities (Puskin, 1992). This barrier is slowly disappearing as more communities benefit from the telecommunications connections between rural and urban communities.

Allina Health System, a managed-care organization based in Minneapolis, has given five rural senior housing facilities the ability to connect with the network for video consultations as well as data exchanges (Kincaid, 1999). In addition, Allina plans to offer these facilities Internet access and e-mail capabilities to facilitate support groups and education for the elderly.

In Kansas, oncologists from an urban, university-based hospital provide oncology care to rural patients using interactive video clinics (Allen et al., 1995). The University of Alaska at Anchorage provides statewide narrow-bandwidth applications serving 4 regional hospitals and 25 remote villages in western Alaska.

Allied health disciplines also benefit from telecommunications. The UCLA School of Dentistry supports consultations with general dentists practicing in remote areas throughout the western United States (Essex, 1998a).

School Telehealth

Kansas and Texas have both developed telehealth applications in elementary schools (Kincaid, 1999; Whitten et al., 1998). With the placement of telehealth units in school nurses' offices, these offices are linked to physicians at universities. Physicians are most commonly consulted for ear, nose, and throat problems. Mandatory school physical examinations and dermatology problems also comprise a large percentage of the consultations. More children are staying in school because they receive healthcare treatment there via telehealth. This translates into monetary benefits for the schools because many systems are dependent for their funding on the number of students who attend on an average daily basis.

Prison Telehealth

Many factors make telehealth attractive as a healthcare delivery modality in correctional facilities. These factors include the constitutional requirement to provide healthcare to prisoners; the growth in, and aging of, the inmate population; the spread of AIDS and other drug-resistant diseases; the predominantly rural locations of prisons; and the high cost and risk of escape in transporting prisoners to hospitals (Essex, 1998a). The University of Texas Medical Branch (UTMB) at Galveston serves over 350 patients per month in its prison telemedicine program (Brown, 1999). UTMB supports interactive video consultations at its 22 prison sites, where the leading clinical specialties, out of 34 offered, are general medicine, surgery, orthopedics, and mental health. The university currently allocates about $1 million annually to fund this part of its telemedicine program.

Emergency Medicine Telehealth

Paramedics have long used a basic form of telehealth, the two-way radio, to provide hospitals with important advance information on incoming patients. Now facilities are installing more sophisticated telehealth technology in ambulances, making a bigger impact in time-sensitive care.

Researchers from the University of Maryland School of Medicine in Baltimore equipped an ambulance with cellular technology to transmit real-time video images and vital signs of patients during transport. The system is being evaluated specifically on its usefulness in speeding the delivery of vital drugs to stroke victims (Thompson, 1997). Studies have shown that the drug tissue plasminogen activator (tPA) can significantly reduce the likelihood of death or disability from stroke if it is administered within 3 hours after the onset of symptoms. Many stroke victims do not realize the seriousness of their condition until several hours have passed, thereby closing the window of opportunity for effective tPA use. The emergency telehealth system provides a ceiling-mounted camera in the ambulance for recording the clinical examination of a potential stroke victim en route to the hospital. The camera can also be removed from the track for close-up views of the patient. The cellular phone then transmits a mini store-and-forward version of the exam at a rate of seven images per second—sufficient for a neurologist to score the patient's gross motor responses. The exam and the patient's real-time vital signs are then uploaded to a university Web site, allowing desktop access for the neurologist. A patient diagnosed with a stroke can be immediately transported to a CT scanner and tPA treatment started within 10 minutes of arrival at the hospital.

North Dakota has 17 counties that qualify as Health Professional Shortage Areas (HPSAs). The Dakota Telemedicine System (DTS) shrinks the distance between rural general practitioners and urban specialists with its interactive telehealth network. Fifteen small community hospitals throughout the state have forged video, voice, and data links with MedCenter One Health Systems, a 216-bed hospital and level II trauma center in Bismarck. Since the project's inception in 1995, MedCenter One physicians have participated in about 200 emergency and trauma teleconsultations, which are 29 percent of their emergency calls. One rural physician called MedCenter One to arrange a teleconsultation with an emergency room physician and a thoracic surgeon when a man arrived at the rural emergency room with a life-threatening collapsed lung. Following the surgeon's directions, the physicians inserted tubes into the patient's chest before placing him in a helicopter bound for Bismarck (Davies, 1997).

Home Care Telehealth

With the continued rise of expenditures for home health, HMOs and home health agencies are investing in telehealth and information technologies to manage costs and service demands. The strategy is to use these technologies to track patient outcomes, reduce service redundancy, and supplement care provided by visiting nurses (Kincaid, 1997). By investing in telehealth strategies, home health providers hope to balance increased efficiency with quality care. Home health telecommunications allow providers to see more patients in less time and to check on them more frequently without numerous in-person visits. Telehealth also has the potential to keep home health patients out of the emergency room and the nursing home.

Kaiser Permanente performed a 1-year study in home care, measuring the use of telecommunications technology for patient access, quality of care, efficiency of service, and patient satisfaction. The participants were 200 patients with conditions ranging from cancer and diabetes to cardiac and lung disease. Monitoring of patients included traditional home visits, phone calls, and video visits using a two-way videophone, blood pressure and pulse monitoring devices, and an electronic stethoscope. The study revealed that using the monitoring devices cost about one-third less than a regular visit, ambulance calls were less frequent, and patient anxiety was reduced (Kincaid, 1997).

A pilot study in Kansas demonstrated that telecommunications enables the terminally ill to remain in their homes. Using interactive video equipment installed in homes, nurses conduct video assessments to determine whether an in-person visit is necessary. This is particularly helpful for rural patients living a long way from the base station (Doolittle et al., 1998).

Research conducted jointly in the United States and the United Kingdom discovered that approximately 45 percent of home nursing visits in the United States could be done via telehealth (Wooten et al., 1998). An example of this cost savings is evident at Boston's Beth Israel Deaconess Medical Center, which uses a home monitoring device that works over the Internet, avoiding the $2000 per day cost of the neonatal intensive care unit monitors for premature babies (Wired Health System, 1998). Evidence of greater efficiency is apparent through a cable television system in Kansas, where nurse practitioners are able to see up to four times as many patients than is possible with in-person home care visits.

The increased quality of the technology and the decreasing cost of equipment are helping to make telehealth an attractive home healthcare delivery option. The average cost of providing a face-to-face home health visit in the late 1990s was $90, whereas the cost of a similar telehealth visit was $20 to $35 (Chaffee, 1999).

ADMINISTRATIVE INITIATIVES

Telecommunications technology reduces meeting and conference costs and increases communication among geographically dispersed administrators. The reduction of costs occurs through bringing people from many distant sites together without travel or lodging expenses or extended time away from their responsibilities. The savings in travel time and costs also encourage people to meet more frequently. Interactions using two-way interactive television are numerous and expanding with time. Videoconferencing is valuable for groups of people at one location who desire to meet with another group at a different location. The audio and video transmissions enable groups of several people to be seen and heard at the same time. Professionals can arrange conferences between different hospital staffs to discuss professional concerns, unusual cases, or risk management. Colleagues can participate in research exchanges through IATV, thus involving more researchers from distant geographic areas. In addition, linking up with manufacturers and computer companies allows direct input into product improvement.

Integrated desktop computing devices are useful for one-to-one audio/video transmissions. Users may sit at their desktop computers to dial up videoconferencing for conducting business. The conference participants can view each other through small windows on the computer screen. Sitting in front of their computers, users speak into built-in microphones. Stored computer files can be accessed from shared workspace and displayed on the main area of the screen. One individual can send a document to another merely by dragging it into a folder icon. If hard copy material needs to be displayed, a user can hold it up to the camera for others to see (Staggers, 1996).

Personal communication devices are receiving increased attention from administrators and practitioners. These devices bridge the gap between cellular phones, pagers, and more traditional computer files. Personal communication devices are portable. They can make phone calls, send faxes, access e-mail, schedule events on a calendar, and transform handwritten notes into word-processed text by tapping an electronic pen on icons.

The administrative benefits of telehealth are closely associated with both clinical and educational initiatives. When making administrative decisions regarding the cost of providing easily accessible, quality care and the cost of staff development, a cost-benefit analysis of telehealth modalities must be considered.

EDUCATIONAL INITIATIVES

Providing education to geographically distant individuals or groups is growing rapidly due to developments in electronic communications technology (Crowley et al., 1995). Telehealth technology is applicable for both professional and patient education. Boston's Beth Israel Deaconess Medical Center uses telehealth technology to offer educational and emotional support to families of high-risk newborns during and after the infants' hospitalization. Parents can watch their baby's hospital care from home on a television monitor and receive guidance from hospital staff after discharge (Chaffee, 1999). A $1.8 million grant from the federal Office for the Advancement of Telehealth enabled a university in Vermont to convert hours of medical and nursing lectures and courses into a multimedia electronic format for viewing by students throughout the New England and northern New York region. The use of this system is increasing for grand rounds and a growing number of continuing medical and allied health education courses (Kincaid, 1999).

To provide healthcare practitioners for a large portion of rural Kansas, nurses started the Kansas Primary Care Nurse Practitioner Program, from which almost 250 nurse practitioners have graduated (Gorman, 1997). Nurse practitioners provide the basic medical care that comprises most of the healthcare needs in the rural areas. Four different nursing schools pooled their resources to make classes available to students all over Kansas using compressed video, a medium that digitizes both visual images and sound and then compresses the information for transmission over high-speed telephone lines to specially configured television sets. Other distance education programs provide classes simultaneously to groups on- and off site, to one or more groups off site, or to individuals off site.

Using one-way video and two-way audio, satellite courses came into existence in the mid-1970s. The video portion is beamed to a satellite and bounced back to the receiving site, and the audio portion is transmitted using telephone lines. Many institutions still use satellite technology even though it has certain problems. Planners must establish transmission times when the satellite is in position. Also, a slight delay occurs in the audio portion of the transmission. Substantial technical support is necessary for satellite distance education.

Since the mid-1980s, IATV has become popular for distance education and is most commonly used today. IATV has interactive capabilities. The instructor can see and hear everyone at each site, and the participants at each site can see and hear not only the instructor, but also the participants at every other site. Interaction can take place at any time. The instructor can answer questions and, at the same time, obtain feedback from the facial expressions of participants. This allows for sharing of ideas and questions that was not possible with previous distance learning technologies.

IATV is delivered through coaxial cable, microwave, or fiberoptic lines. Fiberoptic cable has the most potential for growth because of the large amount of available space on the strands. Many universities, corporations, hospitals, and school systems use fiberoptic cable to transmit continuing education offerings, courses, seminars, and teleconferences.

Even with the advances in technology, the role of the classroom instructor is still paramount in the learning environment. Telepresence is what gives participants in a videoconference the feeling that they are actually in the same room with the instructor. Achieving telepresence is important in telehealth because providers and patients need both verbal and nonverbal cues for a meaningful experience. The placement of the recording camera is important in promoting eye gaze. The direction of a person's gaze usually indicates the focus of his or her interest. If the camera is placed separately from the television monitor, students or patients see the educator looking away from the camera and do not perceive that the focus of attention is on them.

Faculty members must become familiar with the capabilities and use of distance education equipment and plan the course to take advantage of the available media. It is also important to have contingency plans in case technological problems occur. Backup telephone bridges, speakerphones, and fax machines may be used to keep students listening and talking. It is especially important for teachers to plan a wide variety of interactive opportunities and to avoid being incessantly talking heads. Facilitators at remote sites can assist students with small group discussions, demonstrations, critical thinking exercises, and gaming activities.

Each distance education situation requires modifications to the traditional on-campus curriculum and teaching strategies. Administrative issues, adapting the curriculum, adapting to the technology, overcoming the isolation of the student, and evaluating the outcomes of instruction are important challenges.

ADVANTAGES OF TELEHEALTH

With the recent attention to cost containment, managed care, and uneven access to healthcare services, telehealth offers several advantages. Savings can be realized via the following measures (Hebda et al., 1998, p. 251):

- Greater access to care provides earlier treatment for the client, reducing the number of interventions required.
- Treatment can be provided closer to home, often eliminating costly travel and greater urban medical costs. Video consultations between a rural clinic and a specialist can eliminate sometimes prohibitive travel for patients.
- Home monitoring can eliminate unnecessary visits by a nurse to the home or by the client to the emergency room.
- Specialists' advice is more easily accessible, improving the quality of care.
- Physician extenders such as physician assistants and nurse practitioners can provide care in remote locations, with the assurance of physician availability if needed.
- Continuous care is provided through use of local practitioners delivering immediate and follow-up care.
- Videoconferencing opens up new possibilities for continuing education for isolated or rural health practitioners who may not be able to leave a rural practice to take part in professional meetings or educational courses.
- Videoconferencing can also provide education to clients at home and in rural settings.

Telehealth is also a marketing tool. It can foster the impression of technological leadership. It can also expand its market share by penetrating remote markets that are normally inaccessible or too expensive to reach.

BARRIERS TO TELEHEALTH

In spite of the advantages of telehealth, numerous barriers exist. As with other types of electronic record keeping, telehealth's growth has outpaced the development of regulating policies. The safety, security, and confidentiality of the electronic health record are issues for telehealth. Issues that are specific to telehealth include infrastructure, licensing, reimbursement, standards, and patient and practitioner acceptance.

Infrastructure

The infrastructure investment decision is dependent on bandwidth needs and capacity. Image-based telemedicine, especially two-way videoconferencing, often requires leasing of existing high-speed data lines—or the extension of new ones into outlying markets—which can cost thousands of dollars per month. Conversely, standard phone lines and personal computer modems can easily support home monitoring applications, including low-quality full-motion video.

One obstacle to reducing the cost of rural healthcare is the highly variable but generally high cost of the telecommunications infrastructure in rural areas. The Telecommunications Act of 1996 sought to equalize telecommunications charges between rural and urban sites, which could lead to subsidies for carriers and thereby reduce the initial cost.

Many telecommunications companies are jumping on the bandwagon, either providing funding and technology for telehealth programs or improving telecommunications access in many states. These developments should greatly increase the availability of telehealth technology to those who can most benefit from it. Technology manufacturers and telecommunications companies are already vying with each other to produce the low-cost equipment and bandwidth needed. Many states are creating networks to link education, government, business, and healthcare (Brown, 1999). In 1999 both the House of Representatives and the Senate introduced bills to promote access to healthcare services in rural areas (Case Study, 1999).

Licensing

Many states do not allow out-of-state physicians to practice unless they are licensed in that state. In most instances, state licensing laws were drafted decades ago, and the drafters never contemplated the use of advanced communications systems to provide long-distance medical care (Case Study, 1999). When practitioners use telehealth across state lines (or even internationally) to consult on medical decisions, numerous medical licensure questions rise. It is possible that these persons are practicing illegally. Application for licensure in additional states can be lengthy and expensive. State legislatures and state boards of medicine are only now beginning to consider legislative or regulatory changes specifically aimed at telehealth. Some states, such as Arizona, do provide consultation provisions. Arizona allows an out-of-state physician to consult if he or she "engages in actual single or infrequent consultation with a doctor of medicine licensed in this state and if the consultation regards a specific patient or patients" (Case Study, 1999).

To address the question of nursing licensure, which is also issued by individual states, the National Council of State Boards of Nursing, Inc., developed a mutual recognition compact. Although not endorsed by all states, this compact, scheduled for implementation in 2000, allows recognition of a single license by multiple states. Until licensure issues are resolved, however, practitioners providing interstate or international consultations must proceed cautiously.

Reimbursement

Reimbursement for telehealth services remains a difficult issue to resolve but is now being recognized. Legislation in California in 1996 states that insurance companies may not reject reimbursement solely on the grounds that the treatment did not occur face to face (Mullich, 1997). In January 1999, Medicare began reimbursing 745 rural counties designated as HPSAs for telehealth consultations (Chaffee, 1999). Medicare also offers coverage for telehealth services that do not require face-to-face patient care, such as x-ray, electroencephalogram (EEG), and EKG interpretation. Legislation introduced into the Senate in 1999 but not yet voted on at this writing provides reimbursement under Medicare for telehealth services and for other purposes (Federal Telemedicine Legislation, 1999). Slowly, some state Medicaid programs and private insurers are beginning to cover telehealth services. Reimbursement will become a nonissue as programs prove their cost effectiveness and show a return on investment.

Standards

The telehealth community agrees that standards are needed to ensure equipment reliability and interoperability. But there is little consensus on determining the scope of such standards and who should develop them. Most agree that standards should be the result of joint efforts between equipment users and vendors. Different types of data have different needs, so it is unlikely that any one telehealth standard will apply to the multiple modalities in use—from suite-sized videoconferencing systems to desktop store-and-forward units. Varying environments, such as remote locales and home-based services, also create problems. Some standards do exist, such as Digital Imaging and Communications in Medicine (DICOM) for teleradiology and the International Telecommunications Union standards series for teleconferencing and data sharing.

Standards of practice are only now being developed. The American Nurses Association (ANA) developed guidelines to help nurses maintain ethical, legal, and clinical integrity while providing telehealth care (*Box 12-1*). The American College of Radiology also has guidelines in place. Both the AMA and the American Telemedicine Association (ATA) urge medical specialists to adopt standards. ATA has published clinical guidelines for telehomecare, telepathology, and teleradiology (Atmeda.org/index.html, September 28, 1999).

Acceptance

Selling the telehealth concept to healthcare providers and educating them in the use of the technology are often the first major hurdles in a telehealth program. Some providers are uncomfortable using the new technology. Existing referral patterns are disrupted. Territorial behavior may arise as rural general practitioners fear losing patients to big-city doctors or as urban specialists face more competition from other specialists. Physicians and nurses may doubt the technology's effectiveness, or they might be apprehensive about its effect on their own hard-won effectiveness. Having a physician or a nurse, rather than an administrator, champion the program is a vital factor in program acceptance.

Patients are often the biggest proponents of telehealth, but they are not entirely convinced that telehealth is the direction of the future. Two health advocacy organizations, Consumers for Quality Care and Families USA, have expressed concern that telemedicine technologies could too easily replace patient-physician contact, particularly in underserved areas (Kincaid, 1997).

Accepting the technology of telehealth is not difficult; what is at issue is the human factor component and the human interactions. A 1995 study (Whitten & Franken, 1995) shows universal but superficial knowledge of telemedicine by healthcare professionals, appreciation of the value of the technology, but relatively low usage of the available telemedicine service. In this study, the physicians were not afraid of using the technology, but they wanted a more user-friendly environment accommodating the referral practices of potential users. Telemedicine is new to most people, and time is needed to get accustomed to it. An example is

Box 12.1   THE AMERICAN NURSES ASSOCIATION'S CORE
            PRINCIPLES ON TELEHEALTH

1. The basic standards of professional conduct governing each
    health care profession are not altered by the use of telehealth
    technologies to deliver health care, conduct research, or
    provide education. Developed by each profession, these
    standards focus in part on the practitioner's responsibility to
    provide ethical and high quality care.
2. A health care system or health care practitioner cannot use
    telehealth as a vehicle for providing services that are not
    otherwise legally or professionally authorized.
3. Services provided via telehealth must adhere to basic
    assurance of quality and professional health care in
    accordance with each health care discipline's clinical
    standards. Each health care discipline must examine how
    telehealth affects or changes its patterns of care delivery and
    what modifications to existing clinical standards may be
    required.
4. The use of telehealth technologies does not require additional
    licensure.
5. Each health care profession is responsible for developing its
    own processes for ensuring competencies in the delivery of
    health care through the use of telehealth technologies.
6. Practice guidelines and clinical guidelines in the area of
    telehealth should be developed based on empirical evidence,
    when available, and professional consensus among all
    involved health care disciplines. The development of these
    guidelines may include collaboration with government
    agencies.
7. The integrity and therapeutic value of the client-health care
    practitioner relationship should be maintained and not
    diminished by the use of telehealth technology.
8. Confidentiality of client visits, client health records, and the
    integrity of information in a health care information system
    is essential.
9. Documentation requirements for telehealth services must be
    developed that ensure documentation of each client
    encounter with recommendations and treatments,
    communication with other health care providers as
    appropriate and adequate protections for client
    confidentiality.

Box 12.1 (CONTINUED)

10. All clients directly involved in a telehealth encounter must be informed about the process, the attendant risks and benefits, and their rights and responsibilities. Clients must provide adequate informed consent.

11. The safety of clients and practitioners must be ensured. Safe hardware and software, combined with demonstrated user competency, are essential components of safe telehealth practice.

12. A systematic and comprehensive research agenda must be developed and supported by government agencies and health care professions for the ongoing assessment of telehealth services.

Source: American Nurses Association. (1999). *Core principles on telehealth.* Washington, DC: American Nurses Publishing, with permission.

seen in teleradiology, where radiologists must learn how to interpret images using a monitor.

The three basic elements of human factors design—ergonomics, personnel selection and training, and cognitive engineering—are important in telehealth design (Wheeler, 1998). The most important factor in a telehealth design is user input. The end user is most knowledgeable about the ergonomic requirements of the equipment. No matter how technically sophisticated a telehealth system is, if the medical community does not accept it, the system is useless. In telehealth applications, as in other automated applications, it is important to teach people how to use the equipment in unfamiliar environments. Operating a complex system in an unfamiliar environment may affect the validity of an assessment or an interview because the practitioner concentrates more on the equipment than on the patient. The technology must also adapt to the cognitive thinking patterns and workflow of the practitioner.

FUTURE TRENDS

According to Essex (1998b), the most successful telehealth applications have two things in common. First, they rely heavily on information that can be easily seen, such as the facial expressions of people in a training seminar or a particular dermatological rash, or they can be digitized, such as a radiology film or stethoscope sounds. Second, they solve or reduce healthcare delivery problems such as travel time, transportation, and geographic remoteness.

Ongoing telehealth programs viewed as highly successful share certain characteristics. They tend to be well integrated into existing procedures; use existing infrastructure, where possible, to save money and avoid wasteful duplication; and provide an obvious improvement over alternative delivery mechanisms. Suggested future trends in telehealth applications include cardiac care, home telecare, and emergency care.

Telehealth will continue to grow and become common as technical standards and infrastructure, reimbursement, and legal barriers are removed. It will facilitate the move from health maintenance to health promotion and improve the quality of care delivered.

The FCC Advisory Committee on Telecommunications and Health Care calls for an expansion of telehealth applications and recommends the following measures to facilitate its growth (Hebda et al., 1998):

- Higher bandwidth services
- Funding for higher bandwidth services to rural areas
- The creation of a joint advisory committee consisting of representatives of the FDA, FCC, and Department of Health and Human Services to share information related to standards and interoperability of equipment
- The creation of an international working group to promote international telemedicine

SUMMARY

The use of telecommunications to deliver healthcare to distant sites is a burgeoning business. Initially funded through federal and state grants, telehealth applications have become self-sustaining in an era of cost effectiveness, increased access, and outcome measures. Telehealth initiatives fall into three main areas: clinical, academic, and administrative. The telecommunications equipment to support these initiatives ranges from simple POTS to high-speed ATM lines. The advantages of telehealth are numerous. The main obstacles to the growth of telehealth programs include lack of infrastructure; need for interstate licensing; and lack of reimbursement, standards, and acceptance. The barriers are disappearing with the advent of new legislation, and with vendor and state projects to develop and support the practice of telehealth. Increased use of telehealth is seen in the future for all aspects of healthcare delivery and education of professionals.

▶ LEARNING EXERCISES

1. Research the telehealth/telemedicine legislation in your state.
   - Does your state have any legislation regarding licensure, liability, or reimbursement for telehealth consultations?

2. Investigate the availability and cost of ATM, SMDS, and ISDN lines in your area.
3. If possible, find a telehealth site near you and observe the types of telehealth uses.
4. Through a telephone survey of area facilities, including home care, determine if strategic plans include growth in the area of telehealth.
5. Interview a client/patient who accessed healthcare through telecommunications. Were the process and outcome of care satisfactory?
6. Give examples of clinical, administrative, and educational uses of telehealth.
7. Deliver a teaching project for patients using telecommunications technology, if available, or by videotape.
   • How must a presentation be adapted when this delivery method is used?
   • How is the student response evaluated?
8. Observe a videoconference.
   • Was communication free-flowing and effective?
   • Could the body language of participants be observed?

References

Adams, L. N., & Grigsby, R. K. (1995, Fall). The Georgia state telemedicine program: Initiation, design, and plans. *Telemedicine Journal, 1*(3), 227–235.

Allen, A., Hayes, J., Sadasivan, R., Williamson, S. K., & Wittman, C. (1995). A pilot study of the physician acceptance of tele-oncology. *Journal of Telemed Telecare, 1*(1), 34–37.

American Telemedicine Association. (1999). [Online]. Available: http://www.atmeda.org/index.html [1999, September 28].

Auton, S. (1999). *Overview of telemedicine-issues and recommendations*. University of Michigan Health System Telemedicine [Online]. Available: http://www.med.umich.edu/telemedicine [1999, September 9].

Bashshur, R. (1980). *Technology serves the people; the story of a cooperative telemedicine project by NASA, the Indian Health Service and the Papago people*. Washington, DC: Superintendent of Documents, U.S. Government Printing Office.

Bashshur, R., & Lovett, J. (1977). Assessment of telemedicine: Results of the initial experience. *Aviation Space and Environmental Medicine, 48*(1), 65–70.

Brown, N. (1999). *What is telemedicine: Telemedicine coming of age*. Telemedicine Research Center [Online]. Available: http://trc.telemed.org/telemedicine/primer.asp [1999, September 19].

Case Study 2–5: *Interstate licensing*. (1999). [Online]. Arent Fox. Available: http://www.arentfox.com/telemed/telemed_coc.html [1999, September 9].

Chaffee, M. (1999, July). A telehealth odyssey. *American Journal of Nursing, 99*(7), 27–32.

Coiera, E. (1997). *Guide to medical informatics, the Internet and telemedicine*. Oxford: Alden Press.

Crowley, J. R., Russell, B. L., & Martin, S. M. (1995, July/August). Challenges of distance learning for the allied health educator. *Journal of American Health Information Management Association, 66*(7), 61–63.

Davies, P. (1997, October). Delivering emergency care—in a heart beat. *Telemedicine and Telehealth Networks*, 28–32.

Doolittle, G. C., Yaezel, A., Otto, F., & Clemens, C. (1998). Hospice care using home-based telemedicine systems. *Journal of Telemedicine and Telecare, 4*(1), 58–59.

Edlin, M. (1999, August). Get ready for fine-tuning: Telemedicine is on the way. *Managed Healthcare*, 35–39.

Essex, D. (1998a, November). Hop on the bandwidth wagon. *Healthcare Informatics*, 44–52.

Essex, D. (1998b, November). Best apps for telemedicine. *Healthcare Informatics*, 46.

Federal telemedicine legislation, 106th Congress. (1999). [Online]. Arent Fox. Available: http://www.arentfox.com/telemed/federal/106.html [1999, September 8].

Foote, D., Hudson, H., & Parker, E. B. (1976). *Telemedicine in Alaska: The ATS-6 satellite biomedical demonstration.* (NTIS 232/AS). Springfield, VA: U.S. Department of Commerce.

Gorman, C. (1997, Fall Supplement). The wired prairie. *Time*, pp. 61–63.

Hebda, T., Czar, P., & Mascara, C. (1998). *Handbook of informatics for nurses and health care professionals.* Menlo Park, CA: Addison-Wesley.

House, A. M., & Roberts, J. M. (1977). Telemedicine in Canada. *Canadian Medical Association Journal, 117*(4), 386–388.

Kincaid, K. (1997, October). Growing home-care business benefits from telemedicine TLC. *Telemedicine and Telehealth Networks*, 23–26.

Kincaid, K. (1999, August). Hall of Fame members share secrets of success. *Telehealth Magazine*, 30–33.

Lipson, L. R., & Henderson, T. M. (1996, Summer). State initiatives to promote telemedicine. *Journal of Telemedicine, 2*(2), 109–121.

Mullich, J. (1997, August). Hold that line—Get ready for telemedicine. *Healthcare Informatics*, 29–34.

Murphy, R. L., & Bird, K. T. (1974). Telediagnosis: A new community health resource: Observations on the feasibility of telediagnosis based on 1000 patient transactions. *American Journal of Public Health, 64*(2), 113–119.

Office for Advancement of Telehealth Services. (1999). [Online]. Available: http://telehealth.hrsa.gov/services.htm [1999, September 19].

Puskin, D. S. (1992, December 17). Telecommunication in rural america. *Annals of the New York Academy of Sciences, 67*–75.

Schneider, P. (1996). Washington word: Telecom reform. *Healthcare Informatics, 12*(3), 93.

Staggers, N. (1996). Communication technologies for nurse executives. In M. E. C. Mills, C. A. Romano, & B. R. Heller (Eds.), *Information management in nursing and healthcare* (pp. 230–238). Springhouse, PA: Springhouse.

Tabar, P. (1999, September). Smithsonian honors IT innovators. *Healthcare Informatics*, 17–20.

Telemedicine Research Center. (1996, October 9). *History of telemedicine.* Telemedicine Information Exchange [Online]. Available: http://tie.telemed.org/scripts/getpage.pl?client=text&page=history [1999, September 19].

Thompson, T. (1997, October). Taking telemedicine to the streets. *Telemedicine and Telehealth Networks*, 30.

What is telemedicine? (1999, July 7) [Online]. Available: http://208.129.211.51/WhatIsTelemedicine.asp [1999, October 7].

Wheeler, T. (1998, August). Whistling past the graveyard: Don't let your equipment decisions haunt you. *Telemedicine Today,* 10–12.

Whitten, P., Cook, D. J., Shaw, P., Ermer, D., & Goodwin, J. (1998). Telekid care: Bringing health care into schools. *Journal of Telemedicine, 4*(4), 335–343.

Whitten, P., & Franken, E. A. (1995). Telemedicine for patient consultation: Factors affecting use by rural primary-care physicians in Kansas. *Journal of Telemedicine and Telecare, 1*(3), 139–144.

Wired health system: Telemedicine comes of age (1998, August). *Health Care Cost Reengineering Report, 3*(8), 121–123.

Wooten, R., Loane, M., Mair, F., Allen, A., Doolittle, G., Begley, M., McLernan, A., Moutray, M., & Harrisson, S. (1998). A joint U.S.-U.K. study of home telenursing. *Journal of Telemedicine and Telecare, 4*(1), 83–85.

13

Information Becomes Knowledge through Research

Suzan D. Olson

LEARNING OBJECTIVES

By the end of this chapter, you will be able to:
▶ Discuss three broad categories of research conducted in health-care settings
▶ Discuss scales of measurement and measures of central tendency
▶ Discuss how data analytic services can enhance patient outcomes
▶ Discuss computerized applications that can provide analytic support for research activities
▶ Discuss the role of statistical process control in evaluating healthcare outcomes
▶ Discuss ethical issues related to healthcare research

THE INFLUENCE OF SCIENCE ON HEALTHCARE RESEARCH

Florence Nightingale, remembered for her work as a nursing pioneer, has long been recognized as a healthcare researcher. An inquiring mind prompted her to use statistical methods during the Crimean War to determine the incidence of preventable deaths among soldiers (Lipsey, 1998). Later, during the American Civil War, she was consulted on such topics as how long it would take to transport the injured by horse-drawn sled to regional medical facilities.

Today, scientific inquiry and its resultant research activity allows individuals and organizations to formulate and systematically answer questions that improve outcomes, communicate results, and make wide-spread changes to existing systems (Last, 1995). Healthcare research, necessary for enhancing outcomes, integrates mathematics, epidemiology, computer science, information technology, and other analytic sciences.

TYPES OF RESEARCH IN HEALTHCARE

Three broad categories of research are carried out in healthcare organizations: clinical, administrative, and educational research. Within each category, both basic and applied investigations are conducted. **Basic research** has no immediate or practical goal, but it establishes a reservoir of data, theoretical explanations, and concepts that can be utilized in applied research. **Applied research** is aimed at solving specific problems.

Clinical research is carried out in any setting in which patient care is provided and involves examining outcomes relating to those services. Clinical research relies on direct observation, laboratory measurements, survey tools, questionnaires, and other measures. Outcomes include parameters such as improved health, lowered morbidity or mortality, and improvement of abnormal states (such as elevated blood cholesterol level).

An applied research question related to improved clinical outcomes might be: What happens to fasting blood glucose levels when individuals with diabetes mellitus eat a bedtime snack at 9 PM versus 10 PM? Using a software application called a "spreadsheet" (often found on personal computers), participants in the study can be randomly assigned to group A or group B. **Randomization** of participants to study conditions ensures that all participants had an equal chance of being assigned to either condition and allows the results of the study to be generalized to similar populations. Group A eats the snack at 9 PM, and group B eats the snack at 10 PM. Fasting blood glucose levels are measured the following morning. The software program could be used to calculate the average number that represents the blood sugar values for each group. The numbers of the two groups could then be compared to determine if the differences (if any) between groups are statistically significant.

Administrative research is concerned with all aspects of quality, accessibility, and appraisal of healthcare and its delivery (Ray, 1997). It consists of measuring financial outcomes, conducting time-motion studies, performing workflow analysis, or even taking process outcome measurements (see the section "How Research Activities and Statistical Process Control Lead to New Knowledge" later in this chapter). At a minimum, data often used in administrative research include quality indicators, utilization review and case management activities, general trends, and costs of health services.

An example of a question relating to administrative research might be: At what time of the day are patients admitted to a healthcare facility? *Figure 13.1* shows a hypothetical example of average number of admissions by time of day.

As this figure shows, a manager could quickly identify the time of day at which most admissions occur and make decisions about staffing ratios to accommodate the number of admissions. The knowledge gained by such visualization is meaningful in predicting and controlling health care costs.

Educational research investigates the effectiveness of various curricula. The results of such studies can assist educators to devise approaches to clinical teaching and determine the level of practice of graduates from different academic programs. Educational research is conducted using a variety of methodologies, such as direct observation, individual or focus group interviews, surveys, or even questionnaires. These studies assist in determining the effectiveness or value of processes, personnel, and equipment or even the material used in constructing the educational milieu.

An example of a question relating to educational research might be: What are the differences in final exam scores between students enrolled in a self-paced, self-study Internet-based course and students enrolled in a traditional lecture-based course on the same topic? The differences in

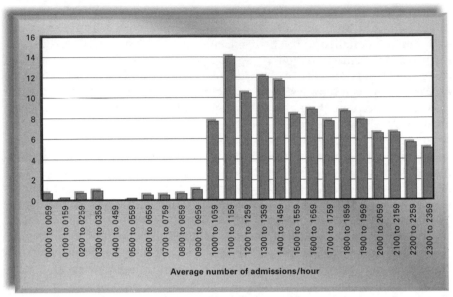

F IGURE 13.1 ▶ Average number of admissions per hour (not based on an actual scenario).

final exam scores could be compared to see whether the students in one course performed better than those in the other course and the statistical significance, if any, determined. If students in the Internet-based course outperformed their traditional-course counterparts, this suggests that under similar conditions a self-paced, self-study Internet-based course might be an optimal way to deliver course content.

HOW DATA ARE COLLECTED

"Data" are raw facts and consist of numbers, letters, or characters— items of information. In order to analyze data, one must first collect good data (Fletcher, 1998). Computer systems are extremely useful in the data collection process because of their ability to rearrange or summarize data for subsequent analysis. However, computers cannot turn bad data into good data. Several conditions are required to input good data into computer systems:

- *Obtain the data legally.* The collection of data should not violate rules of confidentiality regarding patient information.
- *Define each data item.* Clear definitions ensure that current and future users know what each data set represents.
- *Capture the data.* Ensure that all data items are available. Make sure that the entire scope of information is collected.

- *Audit the data*. Before analysis of data can be completed, the data must be audited for quality and completeness. Good data management must ensure that integrity is maintained throughout the process (Fletcher, 1997).

DATA USED FOR ANALYSIS

Data collection is the systematic accumulation of data by direct observation, assessments, questionnaires, interviews, existing records, and even electronic databases. Certain types of data must be recorded in order for the analysis to be meaningful. **Central tendency** refers to numbers that represent the average or typical score obtained from a data set and includes the mean, median, and mode (Kiess, 1996). The **mean** is the average value of the measurements in the data set. It is the most widely used measure of central tendency and has the least variability from sample to sample. For instance, if ten patients provided fasting blood glucose samples for 7 days in a row, the mean (average) value would probably be fairly consistent from day to day. The mean utilizes every value in the sample and is most reflective of the entire set of values being examined. The mean can be used for interval and ratio data, but not nominal or ordinal data sets. (See *Table 13.1* for a description of the differences among various types of measurement scales.)

The **median** is the midpoint of a set of **ordinal**, or ranked, data. Ordinal data refers to data that have been ranked from lowest to highest, from highest to lowest, or placed in some order (first, second, third, and so on). The midpoint is the point above and below which 50 percent of the scores fall in the range of data. The median is not sensitive to all of the values in the data set; the only value of interest is the middle one. Furthermore, the median may not be very consistent from one sample to the next. Socioeconomic data extracted from demographic information would be appropriate data for which the median could be determined.

TABLE 13.1 ▶ TYPES OF MEASUREMENT SCALES

	Nominal	Ordinal	Interval	Ratio
What does the scale tell you about the data being measured?	Quality	Relative quantity	Quantity	Quantity
Is the unit of measurement equal?	No	No	Yes	Yes
Is there an absolute zero?	No	No	No	Yes
Example of the scale of measurement:	Gender: Male Female	Order: First, second, third	Temperature: 98.6°F	Blood glucose value: 80–120 mg/dL

The **mode** is the value that occurs most frequently within a data set. Some data may have more than one mode, or even two or more modes (multimodal). When data are normally distributed, a single mode will be equal to the mean and the median. The mode is the only measure of central tendency that can be used with **nominal** (category/name) data such as gender, race, or type of organization. Its use with numeric data is limited because it is not consistent from one sample to another. Of the three measurements, the mode is used less frequently than either the mean or the median. In examining *Figure 13.1,* it is easy to determine that most admissions occurred from 1100 to 1159. There is only one mode for the data set.

Generally speaking, identifying the type of data to record in healthcare research is one of the first things the researcher must do. From that point on, the researcher can identify the type of statistical analysis that must be performed in order to answer the research question.

DATA MANAGEMENT

The quality of patient care is directly related to the ease and accuracy with which the healthcare professional can enter, retrieve, interpret, and comprehend data (Levine, 1999). Data stored effectively must meet four primary goals: (1) readily available; (2) high in quality and complete; (3) defined in such a manner that they reliably measure what they are intended to measure; and (4) accessible for analysis.

Information in the form of data is stored in a **database**, a collection of files stored as text, voice, or even images. Medical record, laboratory, and medication records might be stored in text files. Autopsy and other dictated records could be stored as voice files. Radiographs, photos, and dermatology and pathology specimens could be stored as image files.

A database is often stored in a **data repository** that contains tools for extraction and manipulation. A repository of laboratory values may be stored in a warehouse containing millions of individual laboratory values (Nussbaum & Ault, 1998). The term **data warehouse** refers to any large accumulation of data. A data warehouse usually contains only a selection of data elements. More specifically, a data warehouse is an enterprisewide database used to support decision making. It is usually located away from the organization and is not generally used for day-to-day operational decision making. Dynamic databases, on the other hand, are used to support ongoing, day-to-day business operations and are usually located within the organization.

"Data analytic services" refers to a variety of activities that transform units of data into knowledge. Corporations use these services to better understand health-related behavior. An example of a service provided by these organizations is **data mining**, which consists of mathematical operations used to identify patterns in data. **Knowledge discov-**

ery, on the other hand, is the process used to extract knowledge from raw data sources (van Bemmel & Musen, 1997). Data mining and knowledge discovery are currently transforming the domain of healthcare for managing patient care, insurance, and financial services. Corporations and healthcare facilities use data analytic services to gain market intelligence, improve business, and initiate new ventures (Barr, 1998; Christiansen & Morris, 1997). Vast quantities of stored patient information are available for analysis and are accessible to agencies such as Medicaid and Medicare, organizations studying aging, the Centers for Disease Control, managed-care organizations, and even pharmaceutical companies (Lillard & Farmer, 1997). Sometimes data are shared as a value-added service. At other times, data are sold.

Analytic services allow "normative database comparisons" (involving criteria used when evaluating healthcare outcomes). Large data sets can be compared, providing information about what is normal, usual, accepted, and even standard. These databases are large enough so that findings reliably predict and describe normal populations. Normative comparisons offer the ability to look at trends in utilization and the cost of diagnoses, procedures, services, pharmaceuticals, and outcomes. These trends can then be compared to local, regional, and national standards of care.

"Disease-specific descriptive modeling" enables an organization to discover trends in patient populations that occur over time. From these trends, relationships between therapies and outcomes can be determined. Modeling analyses prepare the way for decision making and planning that can lead to improvement in patient care and reduction of unnecessary costs.

"Disease-specific predictive modeling" allows information to be extracted so as to combine clinical and business insights with healthcare informatics methodologies and statistical techniques by which to identify relationships between variables. This process allows one to predict future clinical and financial risks and to develop strategies with which to optimize outcomes and reduce risks.

COMPUTERIZED APPLICATIONS FOR ANALYTIC SUPPORT

Healthcare facilities and organizations are being challenged to meet increasing demands for timely, accurate information by taking a look at all decision-making strategies within the organization. The term **health information system** refers to any technology that meets the needs of clinical management. The computer applications found in these systems include database, spreadsheet, and statistical applications, decision-support systems, and expert systems, taking advantage of powerful computer processing to provide needed information. Automated systems for research applications allow the manipulation of dynamic (currently used) or even warehoused data that support diagnostic and treatment effectiveness, patient satisfaction analyses, utilization management, financial outcomes, risk management, and so on.

DATABASES THAT SUPPORT RESEARCH APPLICATIONS

The world's largest relational database is located at the National Library of Medicine (NLM), Bethesda, MD. It provides more than 5 million pieces of information. Many databases located there are freely available to the public via the Internet address http://www.nlm.nih.gov. One such database is MEDLINE. This bibliographic database stores information in a series of tables containing rows and columns so that items that belong together are stored together. The MEDLINE database contains articles describing the results of original healthcare research, but it also contains bibliographic information contained in nonresearch applications, including letters to the editor and editorial comments. MEDLINE stores data such as the author's name, citation, title, abstract, and other indexing terms in a database format. The user queries (asks a question of) the database using these terms to locate a list of citations that contain the search word(s). Bibliographic databases offer the healthcare researcher the opportunity to explore the published literature that supports, repudiates, or otherwise contributes to the advancement of knowledge relative to the topic of interest.

Another large database is the Virginia Henderson International Nursing Library, established in 1980 under the auspices of the Sigma Theta Tau International honor society of nursing. It is located in Indianapolis, Indiana. The Internet address is http://www.nursingsociety.org/library. This repository of nursing research is currently in its third edition. The first edition was a registry of nurse researchers. The second edition was a registry of research studies. The current edition is a registry of nursing knowledge.

The database of the Henderson Library is different from other bibliographic databases such as MEDLINE. It is designed as a source of knowledge about the investigations it stores. Findings are stored as data elements. Only the abstract is stored in narrative form. Researchers register their own work and describe their own studies. They assign index terms, using CINAHL thesaurus taxonomy. Findings are stored in a manner that supports automated modeling of knowledge domains (Box 13.1).

Study findings use as index terms the names of actual variables used in the investigation or the research concept or phenomenon of interest. Abstracts from major research conferences may also be registered and are therefore available for review (Graves, 1997).

Many nonbibliographic databases are also used to conduct healthcare research. For example, HEDIS contains standardized performance measures designed to ensure that the public has the information it needs to compare reliably the performance of managed healthcare plans (McDonald et al., 1997). HEDIS contains data for 1997 and 1998 and includes

Box 13.1   KNOWLEDGE DOMAIN AREAS INDEXED IN THE
            VIRGINIA HENDERSON LIBRARY

- Administration
- Clinical
- Clinical judgment
- Decision making
- Educational

- Ethical
- Historical
- Informatics
- Management
- Methodological

- Philosophical
- Professional issues
- Systems
- Transcultural

approximately 250 plans at this writing. Data include enrollment size, provider turnover rate, outcome measures, women's health, mental health, and access to care, as well as information on member satisfaction.

Medicaid databases provide information on utilization patterns of Medicaid program subscribers. Medicare databases include utilization data for Part A and Part B claims from a representative sample of all Medicare members. The Surveillance, Epidemiology, and End Results (SEER) database contains demographic characteristics, types of treatment, and factors identified as causative agents of certain types of cancer. Information in this database is derived from investigations conducted by the National Cancer Institute.

Secondary data analysis may include data sets obtained from studies in which analysis was not performed by the individual who collected the data. Secondary analysis might be conducted on independent studies taken from the published literature or from population data such as those of the U.S. Bureau of Census. Frequently, data are pooled from a set of randomly controlled trials, none of which is powerful enough to demonstrate statistically significant differences. When those data are combined and statistically analyzed, statistical significance may be obtained. The purpose of using pooled data is to integrate results and identify overall trends. Pooled data from multiple studies (meta-analyses) are often used to evaluate the effectiveness of a treatment protocol and to plan new studies (Last, 1995). In addition, data obtained by secondary analysis can be used by students. In this situation, valuable experience can be gained under conditions that do not expose the patient to risk.

HOW RESEARCH ACTIVITIES AND STATISTICAL PROCESS CONTROL LEAD TO NEW KNOWLEDGE

Human beings have limited capabilities and make errors in predictable ways. The processes that humans use to accomplish everyday tasks may also have deficiencies. As a result, it is not surprising that a recent study showed that 17.7 percent of patients in a major teaching hospital experienced serious errors related to provided services (Andrews et al., 1997; Stahlhut, 1996).

The effectiveness of the healthcare provided must be measured. When deficiencies are found, the causes must be determined and eliminated. These causes may be due to limitations in the performance of individuals or in the design of a process or system. Much medical care is the result of processes involving many people. When the outcome is not good, it may be difficult for an individual to improve it because the difficulties may have arisen somewhere else within the healthcare system. A team approach is needed to understand the process and improve it. For example, clinicians may not act on abnormal laboratory results in a timely fashion. One could blame the nurse or even a resident physician for the problem or the attending physician could blame the laboratory. In reality, the situation is probably much more complicated. A systems approach to process management is paramount to effective healthcare management.

Total quality management (TQM) and **complete quality management (CQM)** are terms used to describe the application of industrial management practices to systematically maintain and improve organizationwide performance. Effectiveness and success are determined and assessed by measuring outcomes. In healthcare organizations, quality assurance traditionally has involved after-the-fact review of healthcare records for adherence to quality indicators (Graham, 1987). TQM and CQM focus on concurrent ongoing analysis of processes. The use of statistical analysis allows the healthcare professional to review, make changes, and track trends over time. As such, quality improvement activities may be measured while the process is occurring. When measures are tracked over time, trends can be identified, problems solved as they occur, and negative outcomes prevented. Through statistical analysis, one can understand process improvement in relation to outcomes. By identifying and managing the link between processes and outcomes, healthcare organizations can meet customers' expectations and play a vital role in improving physiologic, functional, and fiscal outcomes.

In the management of patients, quality may be improved if healthcare personnel use the same techniques and processes for providing patient care. Unnecessary variation may be eliminated through frequent practice and repetition, thereby reducing procedural errors. Improved clinical practice encourages adherence to established protocols, standards of practice, policies, and procedures. For example, Keller (1997) reported on the success of an HMO that reduced average waiting times for outpatient mental health services from 22 to 6 days, and reports of dissatisfaction decreased from 23 to 7 percent. Tamworth Base Hospital in New South Wales, Australia, reported an average length of stay of 21 days for hip and knee replacement. The state average was closer to 17 days. Through process improvement strategies, Tamworth realized a savings of approximately 600 bed days per year, or $200,000 per year (Fahey & Ryan, 1992).

At Intermountain Health Care's LDS Hospital in Salt Lake City, Utah, postsurgical wound infection rates plummeted from 1.8 to 0.4 percent in 6 years through the use of process management techniques. The average postoperative infection added $14,000 to the cost of a hospital stay (Koska, 1992). The reduction in nosocomial infections could reduce the $1 billion a year nationwide cost.

In making each of these improvements, two important objectives were met: improved quality of healthcare and reduced healthcare costs. Both objectives were met through prospective research activities.

ETHICAL ISSUES

The sensitive nature of healthcare privacy demands that computerization protect patient information from exploitation. Security relating to research applications using electronic media has three components: confidentiality, availability, and integrity.

Confidentiality involves protecting the privacy of patients. If confidentiality of information cannot be maintained, trust in science is jeopardized. The potential for litigious activity increases, cash flow may be affected, and future studies within the organization may be compromised.

Availability of patient information refers to the ability of authorized persons to access data. Interestingly, most transfers of nonauthorized access actually take place among authorized users. Unfortunately, access to patient information, or even financial information, is not limited to individuals with a need for primary information, such as those involved in direct patient care. Availability also concerns security—whether the information contained is secure from unauthorized users.

Integrity relates to the protection of data from tampering. It means that data reflect actual findings. When bad data are entered, garbage comes out. In research, findings often result in monetary allocations, potential release of new drugs, and treatment protocols. The release of new drugs and treatment protocols based on inaccurate data could lead to widespread fatalities, with catastrophic implications. Rapid advances in technology will continue to make it easier for researchers to meet growing demands for accountability.

Ethics committees, composed of healthcare professionals and community members, provide forums in which to discuss ethical issues relating to healthcare topics. Committee members generally serve as advisors to health professionals involved in research studies, or to review and evaluate the biomedical and ethical implications of research design.

Over the years, there has been considerable debate about the use of humans (and animals) in clinical trials. Most of these concerns center on the investigator's obligation to participants in the study against the good of society. The factors involved in these discussions include informed consent, the use of placebo therapy, and how participants are randomized to treatment conditions.

The issue of *informed consent* is paramount, requiring thoughtful consideration. Informed consent relates to whether or not potential participants are provided information about what they will be asked to do during the course of the study. They should be told the nature of the experiences they will probably encounter. The purpose of the study should be stated in writing. Informed consent could be compromised in situations in which pressure is applied or when a decision needs to be made in an expedient manner. In any situation, the needs of the patient must outweigh the needs of the experimental investigation under study.

The concern regarding *randomization* of patients to treatment conditions lies in whether or not treatment options are of equal benefit to the patient. If a preferred treatment option exists, then it should be considered. Under this circumstance, ethical concerns do not exist.

Placebo therapy should be considered only if no known therapy for the condition exists. Participants should be informed by the study investigator regarding the probability of being assigned to the placebo therapy group.

SUMMARY

The purpose of this chapter was to introduce research activities commonly conducted in the healthcare domain. The scientific method is at the heart of the pursuit of knowledge. Information systems assist the healthcare professional to conduct scientific research using dynamic data sets or even warehoused data. These applications assist in the manipulation of data for statistical analysis. Automated computing systems thus assist the investigator to transform information into knowledge. Nevertheless, there is no information system today that can replace the sound clinical judgment of a healthcare professional.

▶ LEARNING EXERCISES

1. Identify an Internet-based database available for healthcare research.
2. What type of healthcare research is conducted at a local facility?
   • What databases are used?
   • Is the research process automated?
   • What role does the ethics committee play?
3. Examine a set of data used in healthcare.
   • Determine which data are nominal, ordinal, interval, and ratio.
   • Which data are considered appropriate for the mean, median, and mode?

References

Andrews, L. B., Stocking, C., Krizck, T., Gottlief, L., Krizck, C., Vargish, T., & Siegler, M. (1997). An alternative strategy for studying adverse events in medical care. *Lancet 349*(9048), 309–313.

Barr, C. E. (1998). The role of information technology in disease management: Supporting identification and delivery of best practices. *Disease Management, 1*(3), 121–134.

Christiansen, C. L., & Morris, C. N. (1997). Improving the statistical approach to health care provider profiling. *Annals of Internal Medicine, 127*(8, Pt 2), 764–768.

Fahey, P. P., & Ryan, S. (1992). Quality begins and ends with data. *Quality Progress, 25*(4), 75–79.

Fletcher, D. M. (1997, October). No fool's gold: Guarantee riches from your data mine. *Healthcare Informatics*, 115–118.

Fletcher, D. M. (1998, February). Destination data. *Healthcare Informatics*, 155–157.

Graham, J. (1987, February). Quality gets a closer look. *Modern Health Care*, 20–31.

Graves, J. (1997). The Virginia Henderson International Nursing Library. Resource for nurse administrators. *Nursing Administration Quarterly*, 76–83.

Keller, G. A. (1997). Management for quality: Continuous quality improvement to increase access to outpatient mental health services. *Psychiatric Services, 48*(6), 821–825.

Kiess, H. O. (1996). *Statistical concepts for the behavioral sciences* (2nd ed.). Boston: Allyn & Bacon.

Koska, M. T. (1992). Using CQI methods to lower post-surgical wound infection rate. *Hospitals, 66*(9), 62, 64.

Last, J. M. (Ed.). (1995). *A dictionary of epidemiology* (3rd ed.). New York: Oxford University Press.

Levine, R. (1999, January). Avoid the paper chase. *Healthcare Informatics*, 73–74.

Lillard, L. A., & Farmer, M. M. (1997). Linking Medicare and national survey data. *Annals of Internal Medicine, 127*(8, Pt 2), 691–695.

Lipsey, S. (1998). *Mathmatical education in the life of Florence Nightingale. Biographies of women mathematicians Website* [Online]. Available: http://www.agnesscott.edu/lriddle/women/night_educ.htm [1999, June 12].

McDonald, C. J., Overhage, M., Dexter, P., Takesue, B. Y., & Dwyer, D. M. (1997). A framework for capturing clinical data sets from computerized sources. *Annals of Internal Medicine, 127*(8, Pt 2), 675–682.

Nussbaum, G. M., & Ault, S. P. (1998). The best little data warehouse. *Journal of Healthcare Information Management, 12(4)*, 79–93.

Ray, W. (1997). Policy and program analysis using administrative databases. *Annals of Internal Medicine, 127*(8, Pt 2), 712–718.

Stahlhut, R. W. (1996, Spring). Avoiding the garbage-in → garbage-out phenomenon. *American Medical Student Association Task Force Quarterly*, 22–23.

van Bemmel, J. H., & Musen, M. A. (1997). *Handbook of medical informatics*. Heidelberg: Springer-Verlag.

14

The Future of Informatics

LEARNING OBJECTIVES

By the end of this chapter, you will be able to:
▶ Apply informatics principles and technology to the future of healthcare
▶ Assess how the state of current informatics affects future development

Rifkin (1996) envisions the society of the future enjoying a heightened social conscience that is more humane and ecologically sustainable, not a technological society. He foresees workerless factories, virtual companies, and small teams of entrepreneurs and highly trained professionals controlling events. He predicts that less than 20 percent of the adult population will work full time and that the rest will be paid with redeemable technology tax vouchers. Working with the elderly, children, religion, gardens, and neighborhoods will earn compensation for the tax vouchers. Building the community will be the prized commodity of the future. Those who accept these values and views are, Rifkin says, least vulnerable to replacement by the computer. Digitization and computerization will not replace their skills because caring tasks require intimate relationships between people and are far too complex and difficult to be done by software (Rifkin, 1996).

Perhaps not everyone agrees with Rifkin's view of the new millennium, but without a doubt technology has a tremendous impact on the future of healthcare delivery and practice. Many factors already discussed affect the future development of information processes and technology. Some of those factors are new laws that mandate the protection and distribution of information, globalization of information networking, and lowered cost of technology. Managed care in the United States also affects the outlook of healthcare. This chapter suggests some trends for the future that are progressive and innovative, but with an eye to managed care, based on the ability to:

- Lower costs
- Offer a competitive advantage
- Improve patient care

Future trends include globalization of information technology, increased use of electronic communication and knowledge management, computer modeling and technological advances with the Human Genome Project, use of technology to improve public health, increased use of speech recognition and wireless systems, greater security for automated information, proliferation of telehealth healthcare delivery, and emphasis on the integration of informatics into healthcare curricula.

GLOBALIZATION OF INFORMATION TECHNOLOGY

The **globalization of information technology** in healthcare is necessary and inevitable. Marion Ball, international healthcare informatics expert, addresses the importance of international awareness and partnerships by saying, "The bottom line is we have no choice. We either stand together or we fall" (Schneider, 1998, p. 102). She predicts that healthcare, both in technology and in knowledge, will be a major export of the United States in the coming years. Healthcare technology vendors are broadening their markets to include Europe and Asia. Mergers and acquisitions of overseas companies continue to widen the market potential.

Global networking increases the need to develop a cradle-to-grave electronic health record. Access to new knowledge is also enhanced by global sharing. Determination of a universal patient identifier, standardized system architecture, universal laws protecting the safety and security of patient information, and a standardized healthcare language are all necessary components of global networking on which countries will focus major efforts.

ELECTRONIC COMMUNICATION

Ubiquitous **electronic communication** will surround every aspect of both personal and professional lives of the future. In ubiquitous computing, common everyday devices can and will be augmented by computer technology. The use of e-mail or the Internet will generate no more thought than the use of electricity or the telephone today. Ubiquitous computing brings together a number of independent computing devices to share and update information. In systems of the future, an address added to a personal digital assistant (PDA) also will automatically be added to the desktop system to which the PDA has a wireless connection. Information from a patient monitor will be added to the electronic health record through wireless technology (Turley, 1995, pp. 322–323).

Telephone tag will be a thing of the past, as e-mail has become a more time-effective form of communication than the telephone. Consequently, a physician will be able to respond to questions from more patients in less time. Physicians will create their own Web sites containing answers to frequently asked questions. These sites will contain links to other high-quality consumer health information.

Consultations and the exchange of patient files will take place with the click of a mouse. The security systems that ensure the integrity of online financial transactions will protect the confidentiality of patient information as well. Patient appointments and referrals in nonemergency situations can be handled with the same efficiency as merchandise that can be ordered online. This process is far more satisfactory than dealing with overburdened receptionists who put patients on hold (Grove, 1998).

Healthcare consumers in the future will be much more knowledgeable about their diagnosis, medications, modalities of treatment, and current research because of their use of the Web to gain up-to-date information. They will make decisions about facilities for care and personal practitioners based on Web-published outcome data. Credentials of physicians, nurses, and allied health professionals posted on Web sites will provide consumers with an array of choices for services. Prescription refills and renewals and over-the-counter medications will be ordered via the Web and recorded electronically on the electronic health record.

KNOWLEDGE MANAGEMENT

Data warehouses or repositories are growing in popularity as accurate, timely information, both financial and clinical, as well as business intelligence about markets and customers, become key competitive weapons for decision makers. Because of the trend toward consolidation in the healthcare field, many organizations have massive amounts of data stored in various information systems, but access to the data by users may be difficult. An increasing number of healthcare organizations are realizing the strategic benefit of using data warehouses to tap the data stored in their systems. This emerging information system technology trend is so significant that experts estimate that every healthcare organization will have a data warehouse in place by the year 2002 (Haber, 1997). A data warehouse system extracts data from multiple systems, maps them into a single warehouse, and then accesses and analyzes them at a data mart, a component of the warehouse (Scheese, 1998). This mapping speeds the querying and reporting capabilities of very large databases to provide additional information security or to increase the ability of local facilities to perform detailed transactions at a level that might otherwise be lost in a data warehouse. This information gathering and distribution of intelligence forms the basis of a **knowledge management** framework with a data warehouse at its core. Healthcare organizations that implement data warehousing believe that information is a valuable resource that increases individual, departmental, and organizational performance and productivity. They believe that organizations can use information to competitive advantage, as well as to solve decision support, clinical repository, and systems integration problems. New applications and trends in data warehousing make it one of the most exciting technologies in the marketplace.

The use of data warehouses will speed the dissemination of new knowledge in the future. Knowledge is not static; it is constantly evolving. Fresh insights arise constantly and have to make their way not only to the decision maker, but also into the language used by the decision maker and into information systems (Moehr, 1998). Information systems that support high-quality, complete documentation of care could conceivably derive rules and other forms of knowledge representation automatically. These rules could feed the warehouses of knowledge bases and guide access to patient records, as well as treatment procedures and institutional management decisions. In addition to alleviating the confidentiality problems, information systems could provide a closed loop from care practices to knowledge repositories and knowledge-based decision support. In the future, scientific evidence entered into vast data warehouses could be accessed by all clinical information systems. Entering a patient diagnosis would produce the latest in scientific research, protocols, and clinical paths.

GENOMICS

The large size and complexity of the human genome have limited the identification and functional characterization of the human components that make up the immune system and play a critical role in the front-line defense against invading microorganisms. However, advances in genome analysis, including the development of comprehensive sets of informative genetic markers, improved physical mapping methods, and novel techniques for transcript identification have reduced the obstacles to gene analysis. Technology enables **genomics** and is necessary for genome analysis and application to healthcare. Application of comparative genomics to host resistance will rapidly expand our understanding of human immune defense by facilitating the translation of knowledge acquired through the study of model organisms. The Human Genome Project is an international, publicly funded plan to decipher the DNA makeup of humans. A "rough draft" of the mapping project is expected in 2001, with the project completed in 2005 (Rising R&D Costs, 1999). The final product will assist researchers to discover new disease-related genes and related genetic research.

Genetic linkage maps provide an organizational framework for genes in the genome. Maps, by establishing the location, order, and relative distance of genes, anonymous DNA markers, and biologically important traits along a species' chromosomes, are critical tools in analyzing the genetic contribution to a given disease state. Genetics maps will guide the development of diagnostic tools and drugs that are more precisely tailored to the individual patient.

According to a report by PricewaterhouseCoopers (Rising R&D Costs, 1999), by the year 2005 genomics should be able to create new leads and new areas of business, opening up the markets for diagnostic testing, preventive medicines, follow-up treatments, and even support services such as lifestyle counseling. The report also states that "the genomics industry will see an explosion in the number of leads it can explore, an expansion in the number of conditions requiring treatment, and a growing role within the health care chain" (p. 10). Computer modeling and other emerging technologies will provide the tools with which to locate the best targets, develop the best leads, and test them entirely on screen, dispensing with conventional, expensive preclinical trials and moving straight from the test tube to the patient.

ADVANCES IN PUBLIC HEALTH

One of the major benefactors of the proposed National Information Infrastructure (NII) in the United States is public health. Conceptually, the NII is like a giant electronic web that will allow each user's computer, telephone, and television to connect with others, regardless of their locations or the distance between them, and will enable each user to communicate with everyone else who is connected to the web. Over this network, public and private information sources and data processing utilities will be able to transmit, store, process, and display information in many forms and provide information retrieval and processing services on demand, as if connected in the next room (Lasker et al., 1995), producing enormous **advances in public health**.

Public health focuses on human biology, personal risk behaviors, and hazards on the job and in the environment as they affect the health of individuals and communities. The NII will facilitate partnerships between the public health community and other sectors to identify and make progress toward common information goals that include both policy issues and health information systems projects. It will bring public health, healthcare, research, and informatics groups together to ensure that the privacy of individually identifiable health information is protected in ways that permit critical analytic uses of health data, and that standards for health data meet the needs of the diverse groups that collect and use health information.

Members of the NII project envision a future in which all health-related agencies and organizations are connected to the NII, as are all schools, universities, libraries, businesses, and the majority of homes in the United States. Public health officials will use an array of sophisticated technologies to link, aggregate, analyze, and scan available data to detect changes in community health status and emerging health problems. Information technology will help diverse community groups collaborate on practical strategies for reducing health risks. Disease prevention and health promotion information will be readily available to citizens in schools, libraries, kiosks, and homes.

Parents will receive automated reminders for children's immunizations. Reminders for screening tests based on age and risk factors will be generated to e-mail accounts. One of the benefits of the aggregation of data could be the early identification of potential epidemics. Systems that track identified patterns will alert officials to indicators such as an increase in the purchase of antiemetics in a specific geographic area coupled with an increased number of gastrointestinal upsets reported in physicians' offices and emergency rooms. Street addresses and ZIP codes can pinpoint the incidence of occurrences. The city public health department investigating the problem could use a geographic overlay plat of the addresses of patients and stores reporting increased antiemetic sales from the city's Geographic Information System, which characterizes residents, roads, and public works in different parts of the city. Identifying common sources of water, sewage systems, and food supplies will narrow the investigation and assist in identifying the causative agent. Citizens in the affected area can be alerted electronically and given reporting instructions while clinical alerts are sent to healthcare personnel. This scenario is only one example of how monitoring and improving public health can be greatly enhanced through the use of informatics in the future.

SPEECH RECOGNITION

In the 1998 HIMSS Leadership Survey (Essex, 1999a), the top named technology for the future was continuous speech recognition (CSR). CSR systems have progressed rapidly from the early models that required the person to speak slowly, with distinct, unnatural pauses between words. **Speech recognition** lends itself to any procedure and location where people's hands are not available, such as autopsies, operating rooms, and radiology units, where dictation is already common. Verbally recording assessments and entering orders in a sometimes frenetic emergency room and other settings where the user is either unable or reluctant to type are future applications. Many professionals have been slow to adopt new technologies and the electronic health record because of a reluctance to learn keyboarding skills. CSR bypasses the keyboarding process and allows vocal entry.

The cost savings in such situations are attractive, even though transcriptionists and care providers must still spend time verifying and correcting the output. Although CSR systems may never be flawless, they are about 98 percent accurate, decreasing postediting time. Keeping ambient noise to a minimum and using a high-quality microphone on a special headset increase accuracy.

New systems will record voice messages on a cellular phone-sized device for downloading on desktop personal computers. Two-way conversations will replace the screen-keyboard-mouse interaction of today's systems. Not only will text be dictated, but basic functions currently handled by the operating system, such as loading and closing programs, saving files, and dialing the modem, will be voice activated.

WIRELESS COMPUTING

Mark Braunstein, chairman and CEO of Patient Care Technologies in Atlanta, predicts that in 5 years, more than half of all physicians will use some sort of mobile or wireless clinical application when dealing with patients (Manning, 1999). The devices will be small enough to fit in a pocket for portability. With **wireless computing**, test results can be reviewed, notes taken during patient visits, and references such as drug formularies consulted. A single wireless device can replace the pager, tape recorder, cellular phone, scheduler, and clipboard.

An increase in wireless technology will give more freedom to caregivers providing point-of-care service. They will not be dependent upon a hardwired clinical workstation. Eventually, wireless access to clinical data will move outside the clinic or hospital into communitywide clinical information systems. The incorporation of continuous speech recognition technology with wireless tools is another ambitious goal of the future.

SECURITY

Futurist Watts Wacker has labeled the future the "Age of Access" (Nussbaum, 1999). **Security** not only restricts access but also permits multiple levels of access to authorized users without undue hindrance. In place of the present security systems of passwords—and sometimes multiple passwords—the systems of the future will require only one identifier to grant access to authorized individuals. The identifier is likely to be biometric, such as a fingerprint or a scan of the retina, hands and feet, voice, or face. The use of single sign-on technology will not only substantially reduce the number and variety of passwords a user must master but also, through the use of a dedicated system for authentication, permit greater authentication and ease of administration. Single sign-on systems can also enhance security policy enforcement and central access control log maintenance.

Both federal and state laws will address the specific security needs of electronic information accumulation, storage, sharing, and access. As consumers become increasingly concerned about protection of their privacy, laws on this issue will be enacted. Encryption of electronic information will ensure that an e-mail message, a medical record, or a prescription was sent by the identified, authorized sender and was received and opened by the authorized receiver.

TELEHEALTH

According to the Telemedicine Research Center in Portland, Oregon, **telehealth** consultations have been increasing by a rate of 60 percent annually since 1993 (Essex, 1999b). Although telehealth had a slow start because of high start-up costs and lack of reimbursement, the cost of the technology is decreasing, system capabilities are increasing, and reimbursement is coming. Telehealth of the future will increase the quality of patient outcomes by providing timely consultations with specialists, reducing the trauma, time, and cost of travel for the patient. Prison patients can be effectively served through telehealth by minimizing the security risk of travel and the greater cost of extra guards while providing top-quality specialty care.

Home care will benefit greatly from home monitors for patients that can transmit vital health indicators to a centralized location for continuous assessment. Greater vigilance provided by the monitors on weight, oxygenation, and blood pressure—for example, for patients with congestive heart failure—will result in swift interventions. More timely interventions result in an improved quality of life, reduced hospitalization, and increased patient satisfaction.

The growth of the Internet has given a big boost to telehealth by making long-distance hookups more affordable. Clinics staffed by nurses and PAs in rural and remote areas will enjoy increased access to specialty care through electronic connections to larger facilities. Videoconferencing will become the norm as tiny cameras and inexpensive software become increasingly available.

INFORMATICS EDUCATION

In order to develop a more competent workforce for the emerging markets and to enable students to advance in their professional careers, healthcare education programs are integrating informatics into the educational process. In some instances, **informatics education** is integrated into the overall curriculum; in others, it is a separate course. Often informatics is taught only at the graduate level, but recognition of the crucial and rapidly expanding role of information technology in healthcare and health services management has spurred curriculum reorganization and development throughout higher education.

> The processes and tasks of healthcare, including health sciences education, require extensive use of health information, including its methods, resources, and technology, for diagnosis, treatment, and prevention of diseases, as well as enhanced cost-effectiveness in information storage, retrieval, and use. Inexorably tied to this mission is an increasing responsibility to ensure that our own educational progress efficiently and effectively prepare[s] health professionals who are at once rendered competitive in the marketplace through their advanced knowledge and skills in information management and still imbued with the immense humanity of their tasks.
>
> —Haque & Gibson, 1998, p. 168.

BARRIERS TO INFORMATION TECHNOLOGY IMPLEMENTATION

Although the future seems bright, some major **barriers to information technology** remain to be overcome. These barriers include:

- A lack of nationally uniform policies to protect privacy while permitting critical analytic uses of health data
- A lack of nationally uniform, multipurpose data standards that meet the needs of the diverse groups that record and use health information.
- A healthcare workforce that lacks essential information technology skills
- Organizational, political, and financial issues that make it difficult to integrate information systems into the healthcare delivery system

With the combined efforts of federal, state, and local government policy-making bodies, professional organizations, educational institutions, software vendors, and healthcare institutions, these barriers can be overcome.

SUMMARY

Information technology has become increasingly important in improving healthcare delivery and lowering healthcare costs. As a result, the healthcare environment is going through a fundamental change in terms of the way in which clinical and patient-related information is collected, stored, and shared via electronic interchange of patient records, telehealth, the Web, the Internet, and intranets. In the future, health information will be easier to capture, and laws will be enacted to secure patient privacy and confidentiality. Technology will make information more accessible and comparable across a continuum of care, greatly enhancing the decision-making ability of clinicians and administrators about patient care and improving the ability of patients to make personal decisions about their own health.

▶ LEARNING EXERCISES

1. Write a paper describing your vision for the use of technology in healthcare in the year 2030. Compare it with the paper you wrote after reading Chapter 1.
2. Research the Human Genome Project using the World Wide Web. What is the latest information on the project? What technologies are enabling the research and application of information?
3. Brainstorm additional applications for information technology to reduce health risks. Prepare a visual representation of these technologies.
4. Investigate informatics applications in public health in your state. What future plans does the state have for increased automation of public health information?
5. Visit local healthcare facilities and investigate their use of data repositories. If they are not currently using one, do they plan to do so in the future?

References

Essex, D. (1999a, February). Continuous speech recognition. *Healthcare Informatics*, 84.
Essex, D. (1999b, February). Telemedicine. *Healthcare Informatics*, 100–101.

Grove, A. S. (1998). The X factor. *Journal of the American Medical Association, 15*(380), 1294.

Haber, L. (1997, June 19). Health care industry prescribes IT spending. *Integration Management, 26,* 28.

Haque, S. S., & Gibson, D. M. (1998). Information technology education for health professionals: Opportunities and challenges. *Journal of Allied Health, 27,* 167–172.

Lasker, R. D., Humphries, B. L., & Braithwaite, W. R. (1995). *Making a powerful connection: The health of the public and the national information infrastructure* [Online]. Available: http://www.nlm.nig.gov/research/makingpd.html [1999, April 20].

Manning, J. (1999, February). Wireless computing. *Healthcare Informatics,* 86–87.

Moehr, J. R. (1998). Informatics in the service of health, a look to the future. *Methods of Information in Medicine, 37,* 165–170.

Nussbaum, G. M. (1999, February). Security. *Healthcare Informatics,* 88–92.

Rifkin, J. (1996). The good life in the post-market age. *UTNE Reader,* 56–57.

Rising R&D costs require close management of new technologies. (1999). *Drug Benefit Trends, 11*(1), 9.

Scheese, R. (1998, February). Data warehousing as a healthcare business solution. *Healthcare Financial Management, 52*(2), 56–59.

Schneider, P. (1998, February). Eyeing world healthcare. *Healthcare Informatics,* 95, 102.

Turley, J. P. (1995). Nursing's future: Ubiquitous computing, virtual reality, and augmented reality. In M. J. Ball, K. J. Hannah, S. K. Newbold, & J. V. Douglas (Eds.), *Nursing informatics: Where caring and technology meet* (2nd ed., pp. 320–332). New York: Springer-Verlag.

Glossary

Adjudicate claims: Settle a claims dispute through the judicial system.

Administrative research: Concerned with all aspects of quality, accessibility, and appraisal of healthcare and its delivery.

Adopter categories: Five categories described in Everett Rogers's diffusion-innovation theory of change. The adopter categories are innovator, early adopter, early majority, late majority, and laggard.

Agency for Health Care Policy and Research (AHCPR): A branch of the National Institutes of Health whose mission is "to promote research designed to improve the quality of healthcare, reduce its cost, and broaden access to essential services."

Analysis: Begins by identifying a problem or inefficiency requiring a solution and then determines the best solution.

Analysis of the task: A detailed analysis of all of the activities involved in a task.

Anthropometry: The study of human body measurements.

Applied research: Research designed to solve specific problems.

ARPAnet (Advanced Research Projects Network): A computer network developed by the U.S. Department of Defense in the late 1960s and the forerunner of today's Internet.

Artifacts: Things created by humans for practical use.

ASCII (American Standard Code for Information Interchange): A coding language that translates each character into a numeric form readable by any computer. This universal language allows otherwise incompatible systems to exchange information.

Assessment of the user: The first step in the design and development process; important for gathering information about users and their needs.

Asymmetric information: Refers to a situation in which both sides of an exchange do not have the same facts.

Asynchronous communication: A mode of communication between two parties in which the exchange does not require both to be active participants at the same time (e.g., sending a letter).

Asynchronous Transfer Mode (ATM): A telecommunications method for relaying images, sound, and text simultaneously at very high speeds.

Audit trail: A software tracking system used for data security. An audit trail is attached to a file each time it is opened so that an operator can determine who has accessed a file and when.

Bandwidth: A measurement describing how much information can be transmitted at once through a communications medium.

Basic research: Research that has no immediate or practical goal, yet establishes a reservoir of data, theoretical explanations, and concepts that can be utilized in applied research.

Bedside system: Computer terminal stationed at the patient's bedside.

Benefits management plan: Involves identifying the expected and potential benefits of a new system rather than measuring the present processes.

Biometrics: The statistical analysis of biological observations and phenomena. In the context of this book, it refers to using processes such as fingerprinting and iris scans to create a unique personal identifier.

Bookmark: A software tool that can "memorize" the location of a favorite or often-used page on the World Wide Web. By using the drop-down list of saved bookmarks, a user can return to the page later without retyping its address.

Browser: A software program that interprets documents written in HTML, the main programming language of the World Wide Web. A browser such as Netscape or Microsoft Explorer is required to access the photos, video, and sound elements on a Web page and assists in quick, easy travel throughout the Web.

Bulletin board service (BBS): A computer access service dialed via a modem to send and receive e-mail, participate in newsgroups and lists, or exchange files. Today, many BBSs provide access to the World Wide Web.

Capitation: A payment system in which a caregiver is paid a set amount per patient in advance, regardless of how many procedures are performed later. It is the opposite of a fee-for-service system.

Case management: The creation of a coordinated, ongoing, and personalized strategy for patients who have a variety of healthcare needs, such as the elderly and those with long-term illnesses. A primary care physician acts as a case manager, planning specialist referrals and providing continuity to the separate services delivered.

Central tendency: Numbers that represent the average or typical score obtained from a data set; refers to the mean, median, and mode.

Change manager: A professional who relies on a systematic body of theoretical knowledge to guide the change process; the person or group who initiates, motivates, and implements the change.

Change process: The process of moving from one state to another. In the context of this book, it refers to moving from a paper system to an automated system, from one automated system to another, or from an earlier system to an upgraded system.

Chat rooms: Internet addresses that facilitate online conversations among several users at one time.

Client: A computer connected to a network that does not store all the data or software it uses, but retrieves it across the network from another computer that acts as a server.

Clinical research: Research carried out in any setting in which patient care is provided; involves examining the outcomes of those services.

Cognition: The use of higher-level mental phenomena such as memory, information processing, use of rules and strategies, hypothesis formation, and problem solving.

Cognitive science: A multidisciplinary study of human cognitive processes, including their relationship to technologically embodied models of cognition.

Communications protocol: Rules designed to permit one computer to talk to another.

Complete quality management (CQM): The application of industrial management practices to systematically maintain and improve organizationwide performance. Sometimes referred to as total quality management.

Computer crime: Illegal use of computer hardware and software.

Computer science: Refers primarily to the development, configuration, and architecture of computer hardware and software.

Confidentiality: Respect for the privacy of the information that is disclosed and the ethical use of that information only for the original purpose.

Conversion: The process of replacing an old system with a new one; often referred to as "going live."

Cost/budget analysis: A comparison of the costs of a proposed course of action with its benefits, including both tangible and intangible economic impacts.

Cumulative Index for Nursing and Allied Health Literature (CINAHL): A specialized literature database covering nursing, allied health, alternative health, consumer health, and selected biomedical information resources dating back to 1956. It indexes more than 300 nursing journals and more than 900 journals from all fields covered.

Current procedural terminology (CPT): A procedure identification system that serves as the basis for healthcare billing. CPT coding assigns a five-digit code to each service or procedure provided by a physician. It simplifies billing and protects a patient's medical privacy.

Data: A collection of numbers, characters, or facts that are gathered according to a perceived need for analysis and possible action at a later point in time.

Database: An aggregation of records or other data that is updatable. Databases are used to manage and archive large amounts of information.

Data mining: The comparison and study of large databases in order to discover new data relationships. Mining a clinical database may produce new insights on outcomes, alternate treatments, or effects of treatment on persons of different races and both genders.

Data repository: A database that acts as an information storage facility. Although often used synonymously with "data warehouse," a repository does not have the analysis or querying functionality of a warehouse.

Data security: Protection of data from accidental or intentional disclosure to unauthorized persons and from unauthorized alteration.

Data warehouse: A vast database that stores information, as a data repository does, but goes a step further, allowing users to access data to perform research-oriented analyses.

Diagnostically related groups (DRGs): Patient study groups classified by age, gender, health condition, and predicted treatment needs. A formula is calculated based on the particular DRG to determine how much money providers will be given to cover future procedures and services, primarily for inpatient care.

Disease management: The development of an integrated treatment plan for patients with long-term illnesses or recurring conditions instead of viewing each physician visit as a separate event.

Divided attention: Splitting of attention in several directions at the same time; may occur when one is driving, talking to a passenger, and looking for a street sign all at the same time.

Educational research: Research on the effectiveness of various curricula.

Electronic health record (EHR): Much more than a computerized version of a medical chart, an EHR is a sort of personal electronic library providing access to all resources on a patient's health history and insurance information. It is a linking system rather than an independent database, and is more a process than a product. An EHR can link to separate sources detailing a patient's entire medical history, including images, laboratory results, and drug allergies. The National

Academy of Science Institute of Medicine and the Computer-based Patient Record Institute, among others, have suggested standard characteristics for EHRs, including common coding terminology, clinical decision support, secure confidentiality, and electronic data interchange capabilities.

Epidemiology: The study of the occurrence, distribution, and causes of disease in humanity.

Ethics: The discipline dealing with what is good and bad and with moral duty and obligation. Ethics are the guiding principles of conduct governing an individual or a group.

Evidence-based healthcare: A movement advocating the practice of healthcare according to clinical guidelines, developed to reflect best practices as captured from a meta-analysis of the clinical literature.

Expected benefit: An outcome that the healthcare facility identifies as important to its clinical and business needs, anticipates achieving, and actively pursues.

Fee-for-service: The most common U.S. healthcare payment system. A physician declares his or her own rates and is paid after each medical service delivered; the opposite of a flat-rate plan such as capitation.

File transfer protocol (FTP): A standard application governed by the Transmission Control Protocol/Interworking Protocol for transferring files between computers or across the Internet. Today, nearly every system can accept FTP files.

Focused attention: Attention to one source, excluding all other sources.

Force field theory: Developed by Kurt Lewin, a theory postulating that before a change begins, the forces operating for and against the change should be analyzed. The forces for change are the driving forces, and the forces against change are the restraining forces. The three stages described in the force field theory are unfreezing, moving, and refreezing.

Gateway: A combination of hardware and software used to connect local area networks with larger networks. A firewall is a gateway designed to protect private network resources from outside hackers, network damage, and theft or misuse of information.

Genomics: The study of the human genome.

Good practice checklist: A checklist to assess the availability and accessibility of library services to healthcare professionals.

Healthcare science: The study of healthcare.

Health information system: Any technology that meets the needs of clinical management.

Health maintenance organization (HMO): A health plan that offers a range of services to its members for a prepaid premium. Members pay a fixed rate and usually must use the participating physicians and facilities to qualify for coverage unless an outside referral is approved.

Health Plan Employer Data and Information Set (HEDIS): A set of standardized performance measures designed to ensure that purchasers and consumers have the information they need to reliably compare the performance of managed healthcare plans. Designed by the National Committee for Quality Assurance, HEDIS also is a way for health plans to know what is expected of them.

HTML (HyperText Markup Language): The basic programming language for sites on the World Wide Web. This "skeleton" of codes surrounds blocks of text and/or images and contains all the display commands. A browser program is needed to interpret HTML and turn it into a graphical display on a computer screen.

HTTP (HyperText Transfer Protocol): A language protocol used when Web browsers and Web sites communicate. When "http" appears as part of a site address (called a uniform resource locator), it indicates to Web browsers that "HTML is spoken here."

Human factors: Human abilities, limitations, and characteristics that are relevant to the way in which humans interact with their environment.

Hyperlink: The clickable word, phrase, or icon in a hypertext or hypermedia document that corresponds to a linked page or site. Clicking on the link instantly requests the information available at the new location. Also called a "hotlink."

Hypermedia: Takes the linking concept of hypertext one step further by incorporating linked multimedia elements. Clicking on a word or icon can link to a photograph, full-motion video, or sound clip.

Hypertext: A document containing words or phrases, usually highlighted in a different color, that is electronically linked to text elsewhere. Electronic dictionaries and other software programs use hypertext as a convenient maneuvering tool; users can click on a letter or subject and go directly to the material they want without scrolling through the entire document. Hypertext also is what makes the World Wide Web so valuable: with one click of the mouse, a user can access more information from the same site or from a site halfway around the world.

Informatics: The transformation of clinical data into information, and then into knowledge that supports clinical decision making. This transformation requires an understanding of how clinicians structure decision making and what data are required to support this process.

Information science: The process of sending and receiving messages.

Input: Entering data into a computer or referring to the data already entered.

Integrated Service Digital Network (ISDN): A digital communications route capable of transmitting text, graphics, video, and audio messages at about 64 to 128 K bps. Although an ISDN line is slower than a fiber distributed data interface, it is faster than a standard telephone line and is a popular way to connect local area networks.

Interface: An electronic connection whereby two parts of a system are joined, such as where a software program meets a hardware component or hardware meets an input device. Also used to describe software that joins two different information systems.

International Classification of Disease (ICD): A list that assigns codes to types of illnesses or conditions. Whereas current procedural terminology codes represent procedures and other services, ICD codes represent diagnoses.

Internet: An international network of computers that operates on a backbone system without a true central host computer. Today's Internet links thousands of universities, government institutions, and companies, but when it was created in the 1960s it linked just four computers. Technically, "Internet" and "World Wide Web" are not interchangeable terms; the Web is a child of the Internet whose ease of use has made it much more popular than its less graphical parent.

Internet service provider (ISP): A company that provides modem or network users with access to the Internet and the World Wide Web. Although some ISPs charge by the hour, most offer monthly or yearly flat rates.

Intranet: A member-only network that looks and acts like the World Wide Web. Intranets allow companies to take advantage of Web-based technology and create a private means of exchanging images and text among their networked users.

Knowledge: Synthesized information derived from the interpretation of data that provides a logical basis for making decisions.

Lewin, Kurt: Developer of a theory regarding how individuals adapt to change.

Listserv: A free electronic mailing list service on the Internet that automatically delivers topic-specific newsletters to a subscriber's e-mail address.

Literature database: Body of literature stored in a computing system.

Local area network (LAN): A network of computers and peripherals in close proximity, usually in the same building. A

LAN facilitates high-speed exchange of text, audio, and video data among hundreds of terminals.

Managed care: A healthcare system and ideology based on prepaid membership instead of fee-for-service payment each time service is delivered. Main characteristics: (1) The system usually includes a set group of providers and is associated with a certain health plan. (2) Patients must be enrolled in the relevant health plan and pay the set premium in advance. (3) The health plan and the providers share financial responsibility for care delivery.

Mapping: A process by which the terms used in one information system are associated with comparable terms in another information system, thereby facilitating the exchange of information between the two systems.

Mean: A descriptive statistic that is a measure of central tendency; computed by summing all scores and dividing by the number of subjects.

Median: A descriptive statistic that is a measure of central tendency, representing the exact middle score or value in a distribution of scores. The median is the value above and below which 50 percent of the scores lie.

Medicaid: A joint federal-state program designed to pay for low-income individuals' healthcare.

Medical Subject Headings (MeSH): An alphabetical list of subjects used in a particular database.

Medicare: A federal program of assistance with healthcare costs for over-65 elderly persons and some disabled persons.

Mode: A descriptive statistic that is a measure of central tendency; the score or value that occurs most frequently in a distribution of scores.

Modem: A communication device that transmits data over telephone lines from one computer to another.

Multiplexor: A hardware component used to split a transmission line into subchannels, either by band division or time-sharing, so that several transmissions can travel on the line simultaneously.

National Committee on Quality Assurance (NCQA): A nonprofit organization that acts as a watchdog overseeing the quality of care delivered by managed-care plans and physician organizations. Its accreditation process includes HEDIS and patient satisfaction surveys.

Nominal: The lowest level of measurement that involves the assignment of characteristics to categories (e.g., males, category 1; females, category 2).

Nursing Minimum Data Set (NMDS): A consistent collection of data composed of nursing diagnosis, interventions, and outcomes that attempts to collect data that are comparable across different healthcare settings, to project trends, and to stimulate research.

Optical imaging: Produces an exact likeness of a patient record stored electronically on optical platters.

Ordinal: The amount of a variable placed in order of magnitude along a dimension.

Organizational culture: A combination of beliefs within the organization about the way work should be organized, the way authority should be exercised, and the way people are controlled and rewarded.

Output: Information sent from a computer to some external destination such as a display screen, disk drive, printer, or modem.

Packet switching: A routing method whereby data files are broken down into small blocks called "packets" and sent simultaneously to multiple users on a network. Each packet has ordering instructions so that the receiving system can reassemble the blocks in the proper order. Transmitting a series of small packets usually is faster than sending a large file in its entirety to each user. Also called "fast packet."

Password: An alphanumeric code required for access and use of some computers or information systems to provide security against unauthorized use. It does not appear on the monitor display when it is keyed in.

Personal digital assistant (PDA): A hand-held computer that provides access to notes, phone lists, and schedules, as well as connectivity to paging systems. PDAs have no hard drive, and most lack keyboards. Using Windows CE or a proprietary operating system, input is predominantly pen-based, although speech recognition may become more prevalent.

Plug-in programs: Computer applications designed to support browsers by performing specific tasks. Plug-in programs require the browser to be running.

Point-of-care system: Has a broader meaning than "bedside system," as it includes not only the bedside but also many other points of care in the healthcare environment.

Potential benefit: Any improvement or positive outcome that is possible or likely to occur through the implementation of a clinical information system.

Practice guidelines: An agreed-on set of steps to be taken in the management of a clinical condition.

Preferred provider organization (PPO): A system whereby insurance companies, employers, and other healthcare buyers arrange lower fees with select doctors and facilities. Patients who use a preferred provider pay less, so in theory, the reduction in a provider's fees is balanced by having more patients.

Primary care provider (PCP): A physician who manages a patient's various healthcare services, coordinates referrals, and helps control healthcare costs by screening out unnecessary services. Many health plans insist on the PCP's prior approval for special services or the claim will not be covered. Also known as a "gatekeeper."

Privacy: The right of individuals and organizations to decide for themselves when, how, and to what extent information about them is to be transmitted to others.

Process improvement: An evaluation and restructuring, if necessary, of system functions to make sure that processes are carried out in the most efficient and economical way.

Prospective payment system (PPS): A system of advance payment to a provider or facility for future healthcare services. Capitation is a form of prospective payment.

Prototype testing: Involves iterative or repetitive evaluation of equipment and software throughout the design cycle.

Quality assurance: An assessment of the delivery portion of healthcare plans to make sure that patients are receiving high-quality care when and where they need it. The National Committee for Quality Assurance is a key agency in evaluating the performance of managed-care plans.

Randomization: The assignment of subjects to treatment conditions in a random manner (i.e., in a manner determined by chance alone).

Realized benefit: A positive outcome or improvement in clinical or business operations that has already occurred. It may be an actively pursued benefit or one that is inherent in the implementation of the new system.

Release of information: Generally a form requiring a patient's signature specifying what medical information can be released and to whom.

Request for information (RFI): A letter or brief document sent to vendors that explains the institution's plans for purchasing and installing an information system. Its purpose is to obtain essential information about the capabilities of the vendor and the system in order to eliminate those that cannot meet the organization's basic requirements.

Request for proposal (RFP): A document sent to a vendor that describes the requirements of a potential information system. Its purpose is to solicit proposals from many vendors that describe their ability to meet these requirements.

Rogers, Everett: Developer of the diffusion-innovation theory of change management. He identified five types of people in terms of their response to change: innovators, early adopters, early majority, late majority, and laggards. He also described the three phases and five steps of his theory.

Satisfaction rating: Results of a survey sent to members of a health plan eliciting feedback on the organization's service and quality. The current HEDIS standard requires such surveys as part of performance measurements.

Search engine: A tool for finding information quickly from a variety of sources on the Internet or the World Wide Web. Users can enter keywords or narrow their search using boolean language, and the search engine will list as many relevant sources as it can find. Not all engines are designed the same way; some gather information by keyword registry, and others use a "bot"—a robot program that wanders the Web and scans the first few hundred words of each Web site it encounters.

Security: Protection of information from accidental or intentional access by unauthorized people, from unauthorized modification, and from unauthorized accidental or intentional destruction.

Selective attention: Process of scanning several attention channels at one time in looking for a target.

Skin: Our need to have physical contact and face-to-face interaction with other humans.

SNOMED (Systematized Nomenclature of Medicine): A standardized vocabulary system for medical databases. Current modules contain more than 144,000 terms and are available in at least 12 languages. SNOMED has the potential to become the standard vocabulary for speech recognition system and the electronic health record.

Speech recognition: A computer's ability, through software, to accept spoken words as dictation or to follow voice commands. Vocabulary limitations and recognition abilities can vary greatly from system to system. Also called "voice recognition" and "speech understanding."

Store and forward: A network delivery method that does not use real-time communication. Text or image data are received by the network and held for later delivery. "Later" can be less than a minute or several hours later, depending on the type of communication and the network delivery protocol.

Sustained attention: Limited amount of time that attention can focus on a single subject.

Switched Multimegabit Data Service (SMDS): High-speed telephone lines that are leased monthly at a fixed rate. Also known as "T1 lines."

Synchronous communication: A mode of communication whereby two parties exchange messages across a communication channel at the same time (e.g., telephone).

System evaluation: A comparison of a working system with its requirements to determine how well the requirements are met, to determine the possibilities for growth and improvement, and to preserve the lessons of a computerization project in preparation for future efforts.

System security: Measures taken to keep computer-based information systems safe from unauthorized access and other physical harm.

Systems testing: A multifaceted testing event that evaluates the functionality, performance, and fit of the whole application. System testing includes usability, final requirements, volume and stress, security and controls, recovery, documentation and procedures, and multisite testing.

Taxonomy: A method of classifying a vocabulary of terms for a specific topic according to specific laws or principles.

Telecommunications: Using fibers, wires, radio, and other electromagnetic channels to communicate over a distance.

Teleconferencing: Holding a conference of people at different locations by means of telecommunication devices.

Telehealth: The use of telecommunications equipment and communications networks for transferring healthcare information between participants at different locations. This broad term describes the combined efforts of health telecommunication, information technology, and health education to improve the efficiency and quality of healthcare.

Telemedicine, telenursing, teleradiology, telepathology, teleoncology, teledermatology: Segments of telehealth that focus on the provider aspects of healthcare telecommunications.

Telepresence: Suggests the actual presence of an individual in a room when in fact the presence is virtual.

Total quality management (TQM): The application of industrial management practices to systematically maintain and improve organizationwide performance. Sometimes referred to as "complete quality management."

Transmission Control Protocol/Interworking Protocol (TCP/IP): The most common group of conventional rules for exchanging packets of information among networks, including the Internet. TCP/IP has been used on the Internet since the early 1980s and is considered an international standard.

Two-way interactive television (IATV): Used to connect two geographically distant sites electronically through the real-time use of both audio and visual media.

Uniform resource locator (URL): Like a postal system, every page on the World Wide Web has a unique address, or URL. To visit a Web site, the user simply types the address into the browser program. The URL also reveals whether the site originates from an educational (.edu), corporate (.com), governmental (.gov), or military (.mil) source. Most international sites add a two-character country code.

USENET: An international network of electronic newsgroups accessible through the Internet.

Vendor: Company or corporation that designs, develops, sells, and/or supports a product, which in the context of this book is generally a computer, a peripheral device, or, more often, an entire information system.

Voice recognition: A computer's ability, through software, to accept spoken words as dictation or to follow voice commands. Vocabulary limitations and recognition abilities can vary greatly from system to system.

Workflow: A description of how tasks are done, by whom, in what order, and how quickly. Workflow can be used in the context of electronic systems or people; for example, an electronic workflow system can help automate a physician's personal workflow.

World Wide Web: An international group of databases within the Internet that uses hypertext technology to access text, pictures, and other multimedia with a click of a mouse. Sites on the Web usually are created in HTML, Java, or both languages. A browser program is needed to access multimedia aspects.

WORM (Write Once Read Many): A device that allows the user to write once but read many times (e.g., an optical disk).

Index